MedStudy
Study smarter. Not harder.

Answers

Internal Medicine Answers to Board-Style Questions

Q&A 2

Edited by J. Thomas Cross, Jr., MD, MPH

NOTICE: THESE BOOKS ARE MEANT TO BE USED AS AN ADJUNCT TO THE MEDSTUDY CORE CURRICULUM. THE INTERNAL MEDICINE BOARDS COVER A VAST REALM OF INFORMATION AND A BOARD SIMULATION EXAM ALONE SHOULD NOT BE YOUR ONLY PREPARATION FOR THE BOARDS! FOR A REVIEW OF STUDY TECHNIQUES, READ THE STUDYWISE PAMPHLET THAT COMES WITH THE CORE CURRICULUM. GOOD STUDYING!

This material is edited by J. Thomas Cross, Jr, MD, MPH
Publisher: MedStudy Corporation

MEDSTUDY CORPORATION
800-841-0547

1. Answer: C

The correct answer is he has had a recent MI. Note that he should receive an EGD except that with his recent MI this is a contraindication. His use of ASA is not a contraindication, nor is his platelet count. The attorney issue is left up to your Hippocratic Oath. Other contraindications for an EGD include an uncooperative or combative patient or intestinal perforation—this requires immediate surgical intervention, not an EGD.

2. Answer: A

The answer is ERCP with laparoscopic cholecystectomy. Complications of gallstones include acute cholecystitis, biliary colic, gallstone ileus, fistula formation, porcelain gallbladder caused by calcium and salt deposition in the wall, and stones in the common bile duct, which occurs in up to 10-15% of patients. Occult duct stones remaining after cholecystectomies can occur in up to 1-5% of patients. Rarely, primary stones will occur in the ducts in the setting of increased pigment or congenital abnormalities.

This patient has symptoms of acute cholangitis with Charcot's triad: biliary colic, jaundice, and fever with chills. Many patients with this condition respond rapidly with appropriate supportive measures including antibiotics. The concern is when a complete obstruction of the ductal system occurs, which can lead to severe illness with resulting SIRS (systemic inflammatory response syndrome) or septic shock.

The most appropriate diagnostic study for choledocholithiasis is cholangiography, which usually is accomplished by ERCP with combined laparoscopic cholecystectomy. This reduces the risk of complicated biliary tract disease with the need for choledocholithotomy and T-tube drainage.

One other pearl from this case: If a palpable gallbladder was found (Courvoisier's sign) then this would suggest carcinoma of the pancreas.

3. Answer: B

The answer is barium swallow. REMEMBER: BARIUM SWALLOW IS THE FIRST TEST USUALLY PERFORMED IN THE WORKUP OF DYSPHAGIA. It is done before EGD because of the increased risk of perforation in those with diverticula, and the barium swallow is more cost-effective so it may make EGD unnecessary as in the case of an extrinsic mass lesion seen on the barium swallow. Motility studies are done generally after the barium swallow and the EGD.

4. Answer: D

The correct answer is achalasia. Achalasia may present at any age but usually occurs between the ages of 50 and 60. Regurgitation while bending is common. Usually the regurgitation is NOT associated with heartburn, as is seen with gastroesophageal reflux. Chest pain can occur and in some patients can be severe. Treatment is focused at opening the lower esophageal sphincter. Initially this can be done with pneumatic dilatation with a large balloon inserted within the LES. Surgical intervention via myotomy is also effective. Recently, botulinum toxin has been used, but has a high relapse rate. The barium swallow here was quite helpful in that you can see a large dilated esophagus tapering to a beak-like narrowing at the lower end—the classic finding for achalasia.

Chagas' disease could present this way but you would need something in the travel history to help you. The non-South America clue should have keyed you in to discard this diagnosis. Gastroesophageal reflux could give you these symptoms but the barium swallow is classic for achalasia, and would not be seen with reflux disease. The CXR is also helpful as this is a classic description for this disease too. Esophageal ulcers more commonly present with retrosternal chest pain, odynophagia, or epigastric pain. Acute bleeding could be the only symptom. Again in this patient, ulcer is not likely based on the clinical and X-ray findings. Finally, the Plummer-Vinson syndrome is when you get formation of an ANTERIOR web at the upper end of the esophagus and the x-ray findings do not support this.

---

5. Answer: C

The correct answer is progression is likely to occur and stricture formation with nearly complete loss of peristalsis is seen in later forms of this disease. This woman has scleroderma. Over 80% of patients have involvement of the esophagus. It causes reduced to absent lower esophageal sphincter pressure (unlike achalasia). The other symptoms and signs that she has go along with the disease. The symptoms will not improve as this progresses. Her skin findings are related to her esophageal disease. The gastrointestinal findings frequently involve other areas besides the esophagus.

---

6. Answer: D

The correct answer is pill-induced esophagitis. In adolescents, pill-induced esophagitis is common, especially if they do not take the time to use water to swallow pills. Doxycycline is one of the classic drugs to do this. Other common drugs associated with this include aspirin, non-steroidals such as ibuprofen, iron pills, potassium supplements, and alendronate (for post-menopausal osteoporosis). Scleroderma is very unlikely in a 16-year-old male without other symptoms. Gastroesophageal reflux would not generally cause this type of isolated symptom. Cocaine abuse is not associated with isolated dysphagia. Bulimia could be associated with dysphagia, but he has no other signs or symptoms of this illness.

---

7. Answer: E

The correct answer is improvement with therapeutic trial of anti-GERD medication. All of the findings listed except improvement with therapy should elicit you to get an EGD fairly quickly. They are the "alarm signals."

---

8. Answer: B

The answer is "Because he is healthy, young, and has severe disease that is likely to require long-term medical therapy, surgical intervention with Nissen fundoplication may be his best option. Actually, because he is young and healthy, surgical intervention is likely the best choice. It is unlikely that his GERD will "resolve over time." Because of its side effects (tachyphylaxis, lethargy, extrapyramidal effects, etc.), metoclopramide CANNOT be used long-term. As he has already shown, non-proton pump inhibitors are not likely to be effective. Omeprazole could be used for long-term therapy and is an option; however, because of his age and the documented severity of his disease off of therapy, it will require long-term maintenance therapy, which he may not be willing to do. Additionally, the costs of this drug over time will far out weigh the costs of surgery. The option to see if he improves over time is incorrect because GERD of this severity is unlikely to resolve or improve as he grows older.

---

9. Answer: D

The answer is recommend ablation with photodynamic therapy (using porfimer sodium injection followed by a 630-nm KTP laser applied to the esophageal lumen) Now that he has higher-grade dysplasia, he has 3 options according to the latest guidelines published in 1998 on Barrett's esophagus. The 1st option is standard resectional surgery, the 2nd is ablation, a newer modality, as mentioned in the question with phototherapy (or other available modalities such as cryotherapy, chemical ablation, etc.); the 3rd option is to repeat the endoscopy every 3 months and look for evidence of carcinoma. The ablation method is appealing in that many patients undergoing this method have return of squamous epithelium; although many of these have a deeper layer of columnar epithelium present also. The long-term effects of this therapy are not known and studies are being done to determine if malignancy is truly diminished with this type of therapy. If endoscopy was the only option you would need to do endoscopy on an every 3-month basis. At this stage, decreasing gastric acid concentrations will not reverse the current damage and also, a one-month time interval will not be useful in looking for changes either. Monthly EGD is not cost-effective and very impractical. Finally, application of low-grade beam radiation to the affected area is not indicated and would harm the patient.

10. Answer: A

The correct answer is since she has known *Helicobacter pylori,* it is prudent to treat her with appropriate antimicrobial therapy.

This is a difficult problem. In the first place, she never should have taken the test. The problem is now she has and what to do about the information. We know that in a majority of people *H. pylori* colonizes without causing any disease. Therefore, you would think that because she is asymptomatic further investigation is not indicated or necessary and that no treatment is required. However, *H. pylori* is classified by the World Health Organization International Agency for Research on Cancer as a DEFINITE carcinogen. Here is the problem; Even though it is very unlikely she will ever develop complications from her *H. pylori,* she should receive appropriate therapy. The testing done today is usually quite specific and sensitive for the infection so wasting money on a new test is not likely to be helpful. She is completely asymptomatic and we know that most people with *H. pylori* are asymptomatic so any type of testing such as barium swallow or endoscopy is not indicated.

11. Answer: A

The correct answer is non-invasive testing for *Helicobacter pylori*. In a healthy young person (defined by the American Society of Gastroenterology as being anyone under the age of 45—complain to them if you are over 45!!!), and no "alarm" symptoms/signs, then non-invasive Helicobacter pylori testing is indicated as the risk of gastric carcinoma is low. Indications for early EGD are anorexia, dysphagia, gastrointestinal bleeding (gross or occult), new-onset symptoms in persons ≥ 45, presence of a mass, unexplained anemia, unexplained weight loss, or severe vomiting. Non-invasive testing in symptomatic patients and treatment in those with positive results are cost-effective. Remember barium swallow is the TEST OF CHOICE for dysphagia, not dyspepsia. EGD with biopsy *is* the most specific test for diagnosis of *H. pylori* induced peptic ulcer disease, but is rarely indicated as the initial diagnostic test in uncomplicated ulcer disease in a young healthy person. On the biopsy specimen you can actually look for histological evidence of the little critter (*H. pylori*) or do the rapid urease test on the specimen. Both are very specific for infection if present.

Remember that if this were an older person (>45), then you would proceed to EGD with biopsy of suspicious lesions. So remember under 45..no EGD; over 45…EGD for peptic ulcer workup. Finally, empirical H-2 blocker therapy would be ineffective alone for *H. pylori* infection.

12. Answer: D

The correct answer is "A urea breath test is indicated at this point to determine cure"
About 75% of patients presumed to have uncomplicated peptic ulcer disease due to *H. pylori* infection are cured after one course of therapy. Treatment failure in the remainder of patients usually means that the ulcer will recur. Also, if untreated, these patients are at increased risk of complication such as gastrointestinal hemorrhage. The urea breath test is the best test to assess cure. There is currently also a stool antigen test that is slightly less accurate and its use can be considered if the urea breath test is unavailable.

Repeat EGD is only indicated in certain instances: 1) persistent symptoms after 1-2 courses of therapy; 2) patients with gastric ulcers, or 3) suspicion of gastric cancer.

Cure confirmation can be done at 4-6 weeks after completing therapy. Patients cannot be on proton-pump inhibitors during breath urea testing, as it interferes with the testing. H2-receptor blockers do not interfere with breath testing.

Serologic testing is not effective for follow-up testing. Patients will have positive antibodies for life.

13. Answer: D

The correct answer is serum gastrin level. Several issues should make you think about Zollinger-Ellison syndrome (ZES). Note that his ulcer is in an unusual location; generally any ulcer past the duodenal bulb should make you think about ZES. Also, he has severe esophagitis, which can be seen in regular ulcers, but with the finding of the EGD makes ZES more likely. Additionally, his family history is quite strong and he has been having diarrhea - another hallmark of this syndrome. Although diarrhea often occurs concomitantly with acid peptic disease, it may also occur independent of an ulcer. Etiology of the diarrhea is multifactorial, resulting from marked volume overload to the small bowel, pancreatic enzyme inactivation by acid, and damage of the intestinal epithelial surface by acid. Occasionally you can have mild malabsorption of nutrients and vitamins. The diarrhea may also have a secretory component due to the direct stimulatory effect of gastrin on enterocytes or the co-secretion of additional hormones from the tumor, such as vasoactive intestinal peptide.

Gastric acid hypersecretion is responsible for the signs and symptoms observed in patients with ZES. Peptic ulcer is the most common clinical manifestation, occurring in over 90% of gastrinoma patients. Other clinical situations that should create suspicion of gastrinoma are ulcers refractory to standard medical therapy, ulcer recurrence after acid-reducing surgery, or ulcers presenting with frank complications (bleeding, obstruction, and perforation).

14. Answer: D

The correct answer is alcohol consumption. Note that alcohol consumption is NOT a risk factor for gastric carcinoma. All of the other factors listed are associated with increased risk. Also remember that history of gastric ulcer is NOT associated with increased risk of carcinoma. Other factors listed include diets high in dried, smoked, and salted foods, foods rich in nitrates, and Barrett's esophagus, distal gastrectomy. Uranium mining is listed...so if they have someone who is a Uranium miner look for the possibility of gastric carcinoma. Finally, lower socioeconomic class is associated with increased risk.

15. Answer: E

The correct answer is air contrast barium enema and enteroclysis. She has symptoms consistent with Crohn's disease. A barium enema and enteroclysis will confirm disease location and show evidence of intestinal complications. Lower endoscopy (with or without upper endoscopy) could also be done to confirm the diagnosis. Early in the disease process the barium enema shows thickened folds and aphthous ulcerations. Later, "cobblestoning" from longitudinal and transverse ulcerations most frequently involves the small bowel. As the disease progresses, strictures and fistulas are seen. Skip lesions seen in Crohn's disease. With her prolonged history and initial negative stool testing it is not necessary to repeat ova and parasite testing again. An MRI would be helpful if you were concerned about an abscess but currently her symptoms are fairly mild and no evidence exists for this. Endoscopic laparotomy is invasive and not indicated at this stage of diagnosis. A rectal biopsy is contraindicated and will not provide any helpful information for Crohn's disease.

16. Answer: C

The correct answer is to stop sulfasalazine and use another agent for control of his disease. Sulfasalazine is split into sulfapyridine and mesalamine. The problem is the sulfapyridine can cause reversible infertility in men. The best answer is to stop the sulfasalazine and prescribe another agent or attempt a trial of therapy since he has not had a problem in over 5 years. Once he has achieved "success" then you could restart the sulfasalazine. Formal urologic evaluation is not indicated at this point. Also we have found that his sperm count is abnormally low and this explains why they are not conceiving. His wife does not need to undergo any testing. Also, since we have a reversible cause for his infertility and he is "functioning" properly, it is unnecessary to proceed with further work-up. It wouldn't hurt to try boxers instead of briefs but it is unlikely to make a difference in this case…unless his wife finds them attractive…while his sperm count returns to normal.

17. Answer: D

The correct answer is recommend referral to surgery. Even though he has been doing well until recently, the finding of high-grade dysplasia in flat mucosa indicates that colon cancer is possibly imminent and removal of his complete colon will be curative. It is difficult to think about this in someone who has had relatively mild ulcerative colitis. Additionally, if you had found a mass lesion that showed dysplasia, that would indicate that complete colectomy was indicated. Once you are at this stage, repeat colonoscopy is not helpful and will just prolong the inevitable.

18. Answer: E

The answer is no antibiotic therapy. With uncomplicated Salmonella, gastroenteritis antibiotic therapy is not indicated. If you treated her with antibiotics you risk prolonging her shedding as well as increasing risk of resistance. Remember Shigella you treat; Salmonella you generally don't. Exceptions are the very old, the very young, and the immunocompromised. We treat them with antibiotics because the risk that the Salmonella may disseminate or cause more extensive problems is greater than the risk of prolonged shedding.

19. Answer: E

The answer is none of the choices are correct. Recent information has shown that starting antibiotics in patients with *E. coli* 0157:H7 actually INCREASES the risk of HUS (hemolytic uremic syndrome). Therefore, supportive care is all that is indicated for this patient. Antibiotics are absolutely contraindicated!!

20. Answer: A

The answer is *Campylobacter jejuni*. This patient has classic Guillain-Barré syndrome. Classically this has been described as a syndrome that is spontaneous. However, *Campylobacter* enteritis is linked to about 1/3 of cases. The other organisms listed are not associated with this syndrome. Of note, as in this case, humans can get *Campylobacter* from their pets, especially dogs; conversely, dogs have become infected from their owners with infection.

21. Answer: C

The correct answer is phenolphthalein abuse. Note that she has a normal physical examination and has proceeded past Stage I. The only positive laboratory value is that little sodium hydroxide test, which indicates that she is abusing phenolphthalein. You can also confirm this with specific urine tests for this agent. The bisacodyl could be confirmed also by urine testing. IBS is a diagnosis of exclusion and we have found another etiology for her symptoms. Carcinoid is a rare cause of diarrhea; she does not have any of the other symptoms such as flushing, tachycardia, and explosive diarrhea. Colonoscopy and EGD are reserved for the III stage of work-up of chronic diarrhea and are not indicated at this point, particularly in light of our findings of phenolphthalein abuse.

22. Answer: D

The correct answer is iron deficiency anemia. Remember that iron is almost completely absorbed in the duodenum. With celiac sprue this is one of the main sites of malabsorption. B-12 deficiency is very common with tropical sprue, but not celiac sprue. Folate deficiency is also less likely to be a problem. Celiac sprue exacerbation would not be responsible for anemia of this degree with heme negative stools and no history of blood in the stool. Primary intestinal lymphoma is a rare late complication of celiac sprue—and the key words here are RARE and LATE—so not a concern for this 40-year-old leprechaun at this point.

23. Answer: C

The answer is infection with *Tropheryma whippelii*. This patient has Whipple's disease. Approximately 50% of the patients with Whipple's disease have an associated generalized hyperpigmentation in association with diarrhea, weight loss, arthritis, and lymphadenopathy. Posterior uveitis is seen also. His night blindness is due to vitamin A deficiency from malabsorption—hence the low carotene levels. The clincher was the biopsy of the small intestine and the findings in the lamina propria. Also available from certain labs is a PCR for the organism, which could be used on the biopsy material as well.

24. Answer: C

The correct answer is colonoscopy every 5 years beginning now. A positive family history is the most commonly identified factor that increases the risk of colorectal cancer. This gets confusing a little, so I will break it down in short little paragraphs for you to "digest" easier.

1. Persons with a single first-degree relative with colorectal cancer that was diagnosed after age 60 experience a risk of colorectal cancer at age 40 that is equivalent to that of average risk persons at age 50. Such persons should begin colorectal screening at age 40 (options for this: 1) colonoscopy every 10 years, or 2)annual fecal occult blood test plus flexible sigmoidoscopy every 5 years).

2. People at particularly increased risk are those with 2 or more first-degree relatives with colorectal cancer or a single first-degree relative diagnosed with colorectal cancer under the age of 60 (like Ms. Getalife's dad). The relatives of these affected patients should begin screening at age 40 or 10 years younger than the youngest affected 1st degree relative, whichever comes first. So, based on Ms. Getalife's family history and her dad diagnosed at age 48, she should have started screening at age 38. Screening for these patients should be by colonoscopy at a 3-5 year interval depending on the strength of the family history.

25. Answer: E

No further work-up is the answer. Patients with polyps of less than 0.8cm found on a screening flexible sigmoidoscopy require NO further work-up if they are found to be a hyperplastic polyp. These are quite common and do NOT predict increased prevalence of adenomas in the proximal colon. CEA level is not indicated at all. And the specterfield test is something I just made up for the heck of it because you need something to spice up your life. I hope you didn't run and get on the Web and try and look this up—if you did I'm truly sorry. E-mail me and complain about it. It will give you something to do besides study for 2 seconds <grin>. If you really are upset about this question then please don't e-mail me...E-mail the owner of this company who was stupid enough to hire me.

Luckily for you, the Boards don't do this so if some obscure test is listed it might be something to consider—or completely blow it off too, and pick the simplest test to do—the ABIM is not out to try and trick you. And generally we aren't either, except to add a little levity to your study process. Good luck!!

26. Answer: D

The correct answer is repeat colonoscopy in 3-6 months to be sure that resection was complete. Large sessile polyps (>2cm) usually contain (as his did) villous tissue with a high malignant potential and tend to recur locally after resection. Frequently these lesions cannot be completely or safely excised during colonoscopy and the patient should be referred for primary surgical resection. However, in this case, complete excision was possible or thought possible and it was done at time of colonoscopy. In this case, if a patient has had a successful colonoscopic excision of a large sessile polyp, then he/she should undergo follow-up colonoscopy 3-6 months later to determine whether the resection was complete. If at this point a residual polyp is present, then it should be removed and the completeness of resection documented again within 3-6 months. If 2 or 3 attempts at removing a polyp are not successful, then surgical referral is indicated.

27. Answer: E

Because the incidence of recurrent cancer is small, no other laboratory or imaging studies are indicated for this patient; followup should proceed as with benign adenomas is the correct answer. He meets all of the favorable prognostic criteria by the American College of Gastroenterology:

1. The polyp was completely excised and submitted *in toto* for evaluation.
2. The pathology lab fixed and sectioned the material to accurately determine the depth of invasion, grade of differentiation, and completeness of excision.
3. The cancer is not poorly differentiated.
4. There is no vascular or lymphatic involvement.
5. The margin of excision is not involved.

These patients with favorable prognostic criteria should have follow-up colonoscopy in 3 months to check for residual abnormal tissue at the polypectomy site if the polyp is sessile. After one negative examination, care can revert to standard surveillance as performed for patients with benign adenomas. Because the incidence of recurrent cancer is small, no other follow-up laboratory or imaging studies are indicated.

28. Answer: D

The answer is start adjuvant chemotherapy with 5-FU and levamisole. She has Duke's C colon carcinoma. The spread to the regional lymph nodes is what puts her in that category. Remember that Duke's A is cancer confined only to the mucosa and submucosa and requires surgical removal; Duke's B is cancer confined to the muscularis (B1) or through the serosa (B2) and also only requires surgical intervention. Duke's D is with distant metastases and requires surgical intervention. Adjuvant chemotherapy is ONLY indicated with Duke's C.

29. Answer: B

The correct answer is appendicitis. Right lower quadrant pain with fever should always raise the suspicion for appendicitis. The typical presentation of appendicitis is initial peri-umbilical pain, which then localizes to the right lower quadrant. Fever and leukocytosis are also typical of appendicitis. The presentation of appendicitis in the elderly is often atypical. Pain can be poorly localized or even be absent. Fever may not be present. Leucocytosis is variable. Of patients older than 75 years of age, 80% present with atypical symptoms, as compared with 80% of patients younger than 65 years who present with typical symptoms. The rate of perforation is high in the elderly, because of the delay in making a definite diagnosis of appendicitis. Appendicitis is still largely a clinical diagnosis. Computed tomography with colonic contrast has been reported to be 98% sensitive and 98% specific in experienced hands in diagnosing appendicitis. However, the sensitivity is variable depending on the radiologist, with sensitivity as low as 50%. The addition of intravenous contrast has been reported to increase sensitivity by about 25%.

Crohn's disease is least likely for several reasons. Crohn's disease is more prevalent in whites than in African Americans or Asians. It typically presents at an earlier age, with peak incidence at 15 to 35 years of age. The presentation is usually subacute with recurrent episodes of right lower quadrant abdominal pain, low-grade fever, diarrhea, and possibly a right lower quadrant mass. Acute ileitis, however, may have an abrupt onset with fever, leucocytosis, and abdominal pain. The clinical picture may be indistinguishable from acute appendicitis. Often the final diagnosis is made at laparotomy when characteristic findings indicate Crohn's disease.

Diverticulitis is high on the list of differential diagnoses, especially when the patient has a known history of diverticulosis. Fever, acute onset of abdominal pain, and leucocytosis are consistent with diverticulitis. However, the location of diverticulitis is typically in the left lower quadrant. In the case of redundant sigmoid colon, however, the pain can be located in the right lower quadrant. Diarrhea is often present in diverticulitis. Colon cancer would not present in this fashion and her abdominal pain with the CT findings do not support viral gastroenteritis.

30. Answer: E

The answer is abdominal CT scan. She has known history of diverticulitis (that is what that crazy picture is from 1996) and now with the findings of rebound tenderness and involuntary abdominal rigidity, this indicates the possibility of an abscess or perforation of a diverticulum. Emergent CT scan (or ultrasound) should be done to evaluate for this possibility. Colonoscopy and barium enema should be avoided during the active stage. If an abscess is found then drainage is necessary either with radiologic guidance or surgical intervention. Bowel rest is indicated but you must rule out the possibility of something more severe such as abscess or perforation. A bleeding scan is not indicated as she has no evidence of a severe bleed.

31. Answer: A

Bright red blood on toilet paper in a 25-year-old WM is the answer. The 25-year-old WM likely has hemorrhoids. Everyone else needs a colonoscope. This is a break from all of those long-winded cases. Of course, if you were unlucky enough to get this question as your first question then you have had your "easy" question and life is downhill from here. However, take heart—life might not be fair but MedStudy is (usually).

32. Answer: D

The answer is arteriogram. He has the findings of intestinal angina, also known as chronic mesenteric ischemia. He has the classic triad: abdominal pain after meals, abdominal bruit, and weight loss (from tolerating only small meals). Additionally he smokes and has evidence of peripheral vascular disease (lower extremity findings). He needs an arteriogram to confirm evidence of occlusion in the splanchnic (intestinal) arteries. Treatment is with surgical bypass.

33. Answer: D

The correct answer is hemoperitoneum. He has now developed Cullen's sign, which indicates the possibility of a hemoperitoneum. This indicates severe necrotizing pancreatitis has developed.

34. Answer: D

The correct answer is he has acute hepatitis B and past infection with A. He has acute hepatitis B (he is in the "window" period). He only has IgM antibody to hepatitis B core. He has lost his HBsAg but not developed IgG antibody to hepatitis B core—commonly known as the "window" period. He also has IgG to hepatitis A, which means that he has had an old infection that he recovered from. There is no such thing as "chronic hepatitis A."

On most "screens" for hepatitis, labs do the following tests:
Anti-HAV IgM—looks for acute hepatitis A
HBsAg—looks for acute infection as well as chronic carrier states
Anti-HBc IgM—looks for acute infection in the "window"

Anti-HBc IgG—tells you if a person has been infected with hepatitis B in the past; does not tell you if they are still infectious-this requires the HBsAg test
Hepatitis C antibody: This just tells you if someone has been infected with hepatitis C; it doesn't tell you status of infection (i.e., chronic infected or resolved)

Let's go through the rest of the choices just for fun and how a "screen" would pick this up (come on now...you know you hate this, but it will be on the Boards.)

1) Acute hepatitis A and past infection with hepatitis B: Anti-HAV IgM positive; all of the hepatitis B stuff is negative except hepatitis B Core IgG antibody
2) Chronic A and Acute B: impossible; remember that chronic A does not exist
3) Chronic A and Chronic B: again...impossible for a plain yellow pumpkin...oops, that is from Cinderella, isn't it? Wrong talk about yellow, I guess.

Neither hepatitis A nor hepatitis B; that would mean that all the antibody studies were negative.

---

35. Answer: D

The correct answer is Wilson's disease. The picture is showing you classic Kayser-Fleischer rings, the yellowish-brown discoloration in the cornea close to the limbus. It can present in many ways but a chronic hepatitis-like picture is common. Multiple organs can be involved due to the excess amount of copper. This is an autosomal recessive disorder of copper metabolism. A mutated copper transporting enzyme prevents the excretion of copper detached from the copper-transporting ceruloplasmin into the bile. Rising copper levels inhibit ceruloplasmin formation from apo-ceruloplasmin. A marker for this disease is a low ceruloplasmin but remember that the low ceruloplasmin does NOT cause the disease process, it is the excess copper. By the way, the Cross-Hannaman syndrome does not exist but if it did it would mean you were really cool.

---

36. Answer: A

The correct answer is percutaneous endoscopic gastrostomy (PEG) is appropriate intervention to allow hydration and nutrition. This patient has oropharyngeal dysphagia of which the most common cause is a CVA. There are other neurological causes as well, like ALS. The best study for this is the modified barium swallow. Endoscopy is not helpful at all in our determining the reason for this type of dysphagia. PEG is considered a surgical procedure and antibiotics do reduce the risk of infection afterwards. Other complications would include bowel perforation and local cellulitis. Many patients will still aspirate after the procedure, although this is more commonly due to aspiration of saliva rather than reflux of gastric contents and aspiration of these.

---

37. Answer: A

The correct answer is omeprazole 20mg p.o. ac breakfast. This patient appropriately underwent endoscopy because of his long history of reflux symptoms. Endoscopy is done to make sure there is no presence of Barrett's esophagus, which in this case there was not. He does have significant esophagitis and the issue is what type of treatment gives the most complete acid suppression. Proton pump inhibitors are stronger than the H2 receptor antagonist. However, to fully reach their potential, they should be given before a meal. When given in this way, the proton pump inhibitor will usually suppress acid production for between 12 and 24 hours. The vast majority of patients with gross esophagitis will be found to completely heal with PPI therapy. Sucralfate has not been shown to have significant value in the treatment of reflux esophagitis.

38. Answer: D

The correct answer is reflux esophagitis. Odynophagia usually relates to acute esophageal injury from medications (e.g., doxycycline) or infections like herpes or Candida. Very rarely would reflux esophagitis lead to odynophagia. The appearance above is most consistent with a herpetic infection. Most cases of herpes esophagitis in the otherwise competent host are due to re-activation of a late herpes infection rather than primary infection. These are often brought out by high doses of corticosteroids. Biopsies from the edge of the ulcer are helpful, and the tissue should be sent for culture and histology. These patients may respond even without antiviral therapy, especially if the steroids can be discontinued.

39. Answer: C

The correct answer is 24-hour ambulatory pH probe may reveal abnormal reflux even without typical reflux symptoms. By definition, this patient's motility shows diffuse esophageal spasm, which is characterized by intermittent simultaneous contractions amid normal peristalsis. The upper endoscopy in this case was a very low-yield procedure and probably added little to the management of this patient. However, a 24-hour ambulatory pH probe may reveal that some cases of diffuse esophageal spasm are due to reflux, even if the patient does not have typical reflux symptoms. In these cases the chest pain will resolve with aggressive treatment of the reflux. Some cases of DES will have dysphagia with the chest pain. However, in this case since there is no dysphagia, there is no reason to expect the dilatation would help. Probably the most important aspect of treatment is reassurance of the patient. Nitrates are poorly tolerated on a long-term basis for this. There may be a role for use of calcium channel antagonists, anti-spasm medicines, or tricyclic antidepressants.

40. Answer: C

The correct answer is stomach. Carcinoid rarely affects the stomach.

41. Answer: A

The correct answer is check the stool for *Clostridium difficile* toxin before initiating therapy. This is a case of ulcerative colitis that has developed a secondary *Clostridium difficile* infection. Many flares of disease activity in patients with IBD may be due to *Clostridium difficile*, and this needs to be aggressively considered. In the appropriate setting, the presence of fecal leukocytes would be good evidence of *C. difficile* infection, for instance, in the hospitalized patient who develops diarrhea after antibiotics. However, in the patient with IBD, who may have fecal leukocytes just related to their disease process, this would not be a reliable sign. Many patients, like this one here, will have a leukocytosis associated with *C. difficile*, although this is not specific. Flexible sigmoidoscopy may reveal pseudo-membranes, but is not always diagnostic. Some patients do not have the characteristic pseudo-membranous colitis and in some patients it may be located beyond the range of the flexible sigmoidoscope. In the patient with suspected *C. difficile* colitis, the stool should be sent (preferably 3 specimens) for *C. difficile* toxin. One does not need to send this stool for culture of *C. difficile*. The appropriate therapy is oral metronidazole.

42. Answer: B

The correct answer is amoxicillin-clavulanate 875mg p.o. BID. This is a patient who has scleroderma and related bacterial overgrowth syndrome. Scleroderma has a wide variety of effects in the gastrointestinal tract. They often have severe esophageal disease because of the decreased esophageal peristalsis and the decreased lower esophageal sphincter tone. This leads to severe reflux complications like esophageal stricture and Barrett's esophagus. Decreased gastric peristalsis is also seen. The wide-mouthed small bowel diverticula are characteristic of scleroderma and the bacterial overgrowth is related not only to the diverticula, but also poor peristalsis in the small bowel. The bacteria impairs carbohydrate metabolism, which increases bowel distention. Vitamin deficiency is common in general, although the bacteria can produce Vitamin K, so it's rare to have a coagulopathy secondary to Vitamin K deficiency. The treatment is with broad spectrum antibiotics and many different treatments are available including tetracycline, doxycycline, ciprofloxacin, or amoxicillin-clavulanate. Erythromycin and azithromycin would not be anticipated to help this patient and may even make the diarrhea worse. Metoclopramide might improve her gastric emptying, although this is not causing any symptoms at this time.

43. Answer: A

The correct answer is by attaching a polyethylene glycol moiety to interferon alpha, there is an increased response rate. Interferon Alpha 2a has been the standard therapy for chronic hepatitis C, but treatment has been hampered by its short half-life and wide fluctuations in plasma concentration. A combination of interferon with ribavirin has been shown to have improved results. Likewise, a recent study demonstrating that PEG interferon Alpha 2a (which is the attachment of a polyethylene glycol moiety to the interferon molecule) causes improved results. When compared to standard interferon, the pegylated interferon had a virologic response at 48 weeks on 69% compared to 28% with interferon alone. Likewise, there was also improvement in the sustained normalization of ALT even at 72 weeks (45% vs 25%). Neutropenia and thrombocytopenia can occasionally complicate the treatment of hepatitis with interferon, but it would be uncommon that this would require cessation of therapy. The most common serious adverse effects are the psychiatric effects including severe depression. Factors which would predict a good response to interferon therapy include lower levels of HCV RNA and an HCV genotype other than Type I.

44. Answer: B

The correct answer is paracentesis is the appropriate diagnostic test at this time. Spontaneous bacterial peritonitis is a potentially serious complication of any patient with ascites. Although it is most commonly seen with ascites due to cirrhosis, it can occur when the ascites is due to other causes as well. It may present with abdominal pain, fever, and hepatic encephalopathy, although not all of these symptoms are necessary. The patient may have neither pain nor fever. The risk factors for developing spontaneous bacterial peritonitis include:
1) Prior episodes of SBP.
2) Bilirubin greater than 2.5
3) Fluid protein level less than 1gm/dl
4) Upper GI hemorrhage is also felt to be a risk factor for SBP, and empiric antibiotics are felt to have some prophylactic value. The majority of episodes of SBP are due to enteric gram negative bacteria and non-enterococcal Streptococcus. When performing paracentesis, one should inoculate the fluid directly into culture bottles, both aerobic and anaerobic, at the bedside. An absolute PMN count of greater than 250 confirms SBP. The most appropriate antimicrobial therapy would be cefotaxime 2gm q 6-12 hours. The aminoglycosides demonstrate significant toxicity in cirrhotic patients.

45. Answer: C

The correct answer is transferrin saturation greater than 50% should prompt further evaluation, including HFE gene determination. Hereditary hemochromatosis is a common inherited disorder with a prevalence of 1 in 200 to 1 in 400 populations of northern European descent. It has autosomal recessive pattern of inheritance and the gene for the disease, known as the HFE, has recently been discovered. The patients may present with fatigue, malaise, abdominal pain, arthralgias, and impotence. However, if discovered by screening of family members or screening of asymptomatic individuals, the majority have no complications such as cirrhosis. Physical examination of patients with hemochromatosis may reveal hepatomegaly and skin hyperpigmentation. Serum iron is generally elevated and the iron saturation is greater than 50%. Values such as these should prompt further gene testing. The serum ferritin is usually abnormal, but can be abnormal in other diseases, such as alcoholic liver disease and HCV. If this patient is found to have hereditary hemochromatosis by genetic testing, then he should undergo weekly therapeutic phlebotomy of 500 ml of whole blood until his transferrin saturation is less than 50% and the serum ferritin is less than 50.

46. Answer: D

The correct answer is drug hepatotoxicity. If one includes acetaminophen, then drug hepatotoxicity is clearly the most common cause of acute liver failure in the United States. Acetaminophen is the single most important agent to cause this, although many other drugs may cause this as well. In cases of acetaminophen hepatotoxicity, many of these are due to suicide attempts. However, there are many others who have this due to accidental toxicity during attempts at pain relief. This can occur if the person over several days is ingesting 3-50 gm per day of acetaminophen. Alcoholics seem to be at risk for toxicity even at lower than usual levels of acetaminophen ingestion. Suicide patients often present promptly, but the accidental toxicity patient may have a delayed presentation, and therefore often has higher mortality. If the patient does present early on, then N-acetyl-cystine may be helpful if administered promptly. Some cases do progress to absolute liver failure, which would require transplantation.

47. Answer: A

The correct answer is upper GI small bowel series. This is a 55-year-old with occult GI bleeding that has been severe enough to cause profound anemia that required blood transfusions. No source was found for the bleeding in either the upper or the lower tract. Likely this is due to a small bowel bleeding source. Although it is possible that this could be due to an AV malformation, which is the most common source of small bowel bleeding, he is younger than most patients with this type of bleeding. Therefore, one thinks of other possibilities, which includes tumors of the small bowel, which can present with bleeding. For this indication, one could do either an enteroscopy or an upper GI small bowel series. The x-ray has the advantage of visualizing the entire bowel, although it's not as accurate for the upper region of the jejunum as enteroscopy would be. It is controversial whether estrogen would have helped AV malformation bleeding anyway, and this medicine is very poorly tolerated in men. There is no indication that bleeding rate is rapid enough for a tagged RBC scan to be beneficial. If the GI series demonstrates a tumor in the small bowel, then a CT scan would be appropriate, but not at this point.

48. Answer: D

The correct answer is start patient on iron and monitor the Hgb every 2 months. This gentleman likely was bleeding from the AVM found in the cecum. The diverticulosis which was found was not the cause of the bleeding, as this does not cause occult bleeding. When bleeding occurs from diverticulosis, it is a significant hemorrhage with maroon stool. Likewise, the polyp is too small to cause any bleeding. However, even though the AVM was the likely cause of bleeding, at this point it has not resulted in significant blood loss such that the patient is asymptomatic. It is likely that this patient can be placed on iron and his Hgb will stabilize. He may slowly ooze blood from time to time, but the iron will replace those losses. Estrogen therapy is not of proven value for AV malformations and it's not tolerated by men because of the side effects.

49. Answer: C

The correct answer is this patient will likely not have recurrent bleeding after admission, though his Hct will likely fall with hydration. This patient does have bleeding from a Mallory-Weiss tear, and it is often the case that the patient does not remember prior retching. However, given that there is no fresh blood in the stomach, no oozing from the linear tear, or visible vessel, he does have a favorable prognosis as far as the bleeding has likely stopped. There is no indication for endoscopic therapy unless there is active bleeding or a visible vessel. Mallory-Weiss tears can certainly be a cause of massive hemorrhage, although not in this case above.

50. Answer: D

The correct answer is admission to an observation unit with Hct every 4 hours and discharge the next day if stable. This patient has developed a duodenal ulcer probably due to the daily aspirin intake. However, the bleeding stopped several days ago and with the endoscopic picture showing a clean base, there is very little likelihood of further bleeding. Her risk of rebleeding at this point is between 0 and 5%. At this point, it is very safe to let her go home on oral therapy for the ulcer. She needs to be advised to avoid aspirin. There is no value to endoscopic treatment in this patient, which would only be indicated if there was a visible vessel or active bleeding.

51. Answer: C

The correct answer is colonoscopy and endoscopy. If the latter is grossly normal, obtain oriented biopsies of the duodenum. The patient has celiac disease. This has led to the bloating and loose stools, which represent malabsorption, as well as her iron deficiency anemia. The iron deficiency anemia may not be due to occult bleeding, but rather interference with the absorption of iron, which takes place mainly in the duodenum. The duodenum is the region in the small bowel most affected by celiac disease and it is not uncommon for these patients to be iron deficient. However, performing a colonoscopy and endoscopy is correct because in her age group, a full endoscopic evaluation needs to be done on anybody with an iron deficiency anemia, even in the absence of heme positive stools. Clearly colonoscopy needs to be done to rule out colon cancer. On upper exam, there are some characteristic findings that can indicate celiac disease. The duodenal folds may be atrophic or have a scalloped appearance. However, even in the absence of endoscopic findings, one should do the oriented biopsies of the duodenum if one suspects celiac disease. The upper GI series would not be accurate enough to show any specific changes for celiac disease. The antigliadin and antiendomysial antibodies can be helpful in diagnosing patients with celiac disease, but the gold standard of diagnosis stills relies on duodenal biopsies and one should have that before making the diagnosis and initiating therapy. In this case, one would simply treat with a gluten-free diet, saving steroids for more difficult and refractory cases.

52. Answer: B

The correct answer is ERCP. This patient with ulcerative colitis has likely developed primary sclerosing cholangitis. Of all patients with PSC, 70% will have a history of ulcerative colitis. Just like in the case of this patient, there is a strong male predominance. Many of these patients are asymptomatic at the onset. Some will give symptoms of cholangitis, such as fever and chills, and some may present with fatigue and malaise. At the time of ERCP, there may be multiple strictures of both the intra and extrahepatic bile ducts. There often is not enough dilatation for this to be noted on studies such as the ultrasound. Dominant strictures of the bile duct can be dilated at the time of ERCP. There is no additional value to a liver biopsy at this time. An abdominal CT scan would likely not add any more than the ultrasound already did. And finally, there is no indication for laparoscopic cholecystectomy either.

53. Answer: A

The correct answer is ERCP now, since there is a high likelihood of stones present in the CBD. This woman has had a case of pancreatitis likely secondary to a passed gallstone. Although the ultrasound did not show any stone or stones in the common duct or dilatation in the common duct, there are several factors here that would predict a moderate possibility of persistent stones in the duct. This would be the fact that her laboratories increased on the day after admission and also the fact that her bilirubin went as high as 3.5. Therefore, with this moderate possibility of retained stones in the CBD, an ERCP is reasonable. ERCP does not necessarily have to be done before cholecystectomy. Some would say do a laparoscopic cholecystectomy with an intraoperative cholangiogram, and then proceed with an ERCP after surgery if the cholangiogram is positive for stones. However, this is a case where it is probably appropriate to do the study preoperatively. There is no value in sending the patient home before coming back to have surgery in this case, since her abdomen is completely benign. Likewise, there is no reason why she can't have a laparoscopic cholecystectomy, as there is no need for the increased morbidity associated with the open procedure with common duct exploration. Although percutaneous cholangiogram will clearly identify stones in the common duct, it does not have the same therapeutic potential of being able to remove the stones readily that an ERCP does.

54. Answer: C

The correct answer is consult Surgery for elective resection of the tail of the pancreas with removal of the cyst. This patient does indeed have a cyst of the pancreas, but it is unlikely that this is a pseudocyst, given that she has never had pain or symptoms to suggest either acute or chronic pancreatitis. In this case, one must consider the possibility of a cystic neoplasm, which can be either a cystadenoma or a cystadenocarcinoma or, rarely, cystic islet cell tumors. A CA19-9 level might be elevated in cases of pancreatic adenocarcinoma, but it would not be helpful in the cystic neoplasms. Likewise, CT-directed needle aspiration often yields negative cytology even in the case of cystadenocarcinoma. Since this lady is healthy, she should undergo resection of the tail of the pancreas, which is a relatively easy procedure and will be curative in this case.

55. Answer: B

The correct answer is this is likely a *Staphylococcus aureus* food poisoning. These patients have the typical description of *Staph aureus* food poisoning. Patients usually present 4-6 hours after ingestion of the food with nausea, vomiting, and diarrhea. These symptoms do not last long, rarely more than 12 hours, but it is not uncommon to have severe dehydration. The *Staph aureus* could have been obtained in the ham or even the deviled eggs. Although undercooked poultry can be a source of *Salmonella*, the incubation period is much longer than what is seen here. Likewise, in *E. coli* 0157, the incubation period is longer as well. Giardiasis can occur after ingesting Rocky Mountain water, but the symptoms are too severe in this case.

The treatment of *Staph aureus* food poisoning revolves around supportive intravenous fluid. This is an ingested toxin rather than any active bacteria, so there is no value in giving antibiotics.

56. Answer: B

The answer is carbon monoxide poisoning. All of the workers were diagnosed as suffering from carbon monoxide poisoning. CO has been called the silent killer and is the cause of approximately 5,000 deaths annually, with 2 to 5 times that number requiring treatment. Even with treatment, the devastating sequelae that can accompany CO poisoning can be life changing. These include chorea, rigidity, dementia, myoclonus, impaired sensory function, seizures, and gait dysfunction. There can also be permanent cardiac damage due to the hypoxia involved in the poisoning process.

CO is an odorless, colorless, and tasteless gas that results from incomplete combustion of fuels (i.e., coal, wood, gasoline). Once inhaled it binds quickly and tightly to the hemoglobin (Hgb), crowds out the oxygen, and studies have shown CO can bind 200 times stronger than oxygen. Since the Hgb can no longer carry the oxygen the patient becomes hypoxemic and anoxic. Also, the CO binds with myoglobin in the muscles and interferes with cellular metabolism, causing metabolic acidosis.

Normal carboxyhemoglobin (HbCO) levels are 0-3% for nonsmokers and 3-8% for smokers. A level of 10-20% causes headaches, nausea, vomiting, and dyspnea. A level of 30-40% causes severe headaches, syncope, and tachyarrhythmias. Greater than 40% causes Cheyne-Stokes respiration or respiratory failure, seizures, unconsciousness, permanent brain damage, cardiac arrest, and even death.

Because of the vagueness of the symptoms and their similarity to flu-like symptoms (nausea, vomiting, dizziness, headache, etc.) CO poisoning is often misdiagnosed. Also, even if HbCO is present it cannot be diagnosed with a simple pulse oximetry device because the displayed saturation level equals the sum of the oxyhemoglobin and carboxyhemoglobin.

So if a patient comes to you and CO poisoning is suspected, what should you do? First and foremost, the patient needs high flow, high concentration O_2, preferably a non-rebreather mask at 15 liters per minute, as well as a large bore IV. Prepare for blood draws (ABG, CBC, Lytes, CPK, Lactate, and Carboxyhemoglobin); a urine sample is also useful to rule out rhabdomyolysis (cardiac muscle breakdown secondary to the myoglobin damage from CO). Other treatment modalities may include a CXR, cardiac monitoring, and possibly Mannitol (1-2G/kg) to help decrease the cerebral edema accompanying the CO poisoning. Finally, probably the most effective treatment is transfer of the patient to a hyperbaric oxygen unit (HBO). This is clearly indicated when the patient is very symptomatic and/or the HbCO is 25% or greater.

57. Answer: D

The correct answer is Ciprofloxacin. The problem is that he is on theophylline and adding ciprofloxacin has caused his theophylline clearance to decrease, thus resulting in increased serum levels of theophylline. The result of increased theophylline levels in the toxic range usually begins with nausea and vomiting. The other antibiotics do not induce changes in theophylline clearance. (Oh yeah, astringimycin is not a real antibiotic so don't worry about having to go learn a whole new class of antibiotics.)

58. Answer: D

The answer is low rate, small tidal volume, and high flows. When ventilating an asthmatic patient, the idea of "permissive hypercapnia" is important to remember. Focus on getting the oxygen saturation up and don't worry as much about the pCO_2. Each of the factors (low rate, small tidal volume, high flows) addresses the need for a prolonged expiratory phase. High flow on the inspiration allows for less time devoted to inspiration and more time to expiration. So, based on the idea of "permissive hypercapnia," it makes sense to have a lower rate and smaller tidal volume.

59. Answer: C

The answer is supplemental oxygen should be worn 24 hours a day by this patient. Only objective data from an arterial blood gas is acceptable to Medicare agents for supplemental oxygen. History and physical examination will not help get this funded. He needs to meet one of the following criteria:

1. resting $PaO_2 < 55$ mm Hg, OR
2. O_2 saturation $\leq 88\%$, OR
3. $PaO_2 < 59$ mm Hg (O_2 sat $\geq 89\%$) with evidence of cor pulmonale or erythrocytosis (hematocrit > 55%).

You can tell him that being on supplemental oxygen is likely to improve his symptoms and there is a possibility that in several months he may not need the oxygen anymore. Therefore, you need to bring him back in 2 months and retest him. Note that the use of supplemental oxygen does NOT depress the respiratory drive and cause an elevated CO_2. It is due to several factors, including an easing of pulmonary vasoconstriction, which leads to perfusion of previously unperfused spaces and possibly due to ventilation of previous dead space.

60. Answer: D

The answer is family history. It would be exceedingly unusual for a male patient with cystic fibrosis to have children. The rest of the findings are consistent with CF. Remember that this gene is encoded on Chromosome 7. It causes a defect in sodium and chloride transport channels in lungs particularly, but also in other organs.

61. Answer: D

Of the answers listed, the one that would NOT be an indication of removing mechanical ventilation is having a PEEP of 10 cm H_2O. PEEP should be less than 5 cm H_2O before discontinuation of mechanical ventilation and extubation can be considered. Vital capacity should be greater than 10 to 15 ml/kg. Tidal volume of 4 to 5 ml/kg is acceptable for removal from the ventilator. FiO_2 should be less than 40% before discontinuation of mechanical ventilation. $P(A-a)O_2$ at an FiO_2 of 100%, less than 350 mm Hg for successful weaning off the ventilator and extubation.

62. Answer: D

Silicosis

The correct answer is Start INH prophylaxis. This patient has silicosis based on his history of working in a brickyard and the classic findings on CXR of small nodules in the upper lobes that are calcified and the "hilar eggshell calcifications". There is no specific treatment for uncomplicated silicosis. The problem with silicosis,

Also - exposure to close contact > 5 mm treat

however, is that alveolar macrophages are made ineffective by the ingestion of silica, therefore patients with silicosis are at increased risk of tuberculosis. Therefore, anytime a patient with known silicosis has a positive PPD no matter what age or duration, they should be prophylaxed with INH. He has no evidence of active disease and therefore treatment with 4-drug therapy is not indicated. Asbestosis more commonly involves the lower lobes and his presentation does not warrant a big work-up for this disease.

---

63. Answer: D

The answer is Langerhans cells. This patient most likely has eosinophilic granuloma. Langerhans cells are the predominant cell form. It occurs in smokers and men much more often than women. About 10% of patients will present with pneumothorax.

The diabetes insipidus is seen when the granuloma involve the posterior pituitary. Treatment is to STOP SMOKING. If he had lytic bone lesions (particularly skull), diabetes insipidus, and exophthalmus, then he would have Hand-Schüller-Christian syndrome.

---

64. Answer: A

This patient has classic findings of pulmonary sarcoidosis. Her chest radiograph shows a diffuse miliary pattern, which is suspicious for tuberculous or metastatic carcinoma. Her biopsy shows two small, non-necrotizing granulomas. The differential diagnosis includes mainly infectious granulomatous disease, hypersensitivity pneumonia, and sarcoidosis. Granulomas may also be seen with aspiration pneumonia, in chronic beryllium disease or exposure to titanium or aluminum dusts, as a response to certain drugs, and rarely with Wegener's granulomatosis, lymphocytic interstitial pneumonia or eosinophilic pneumonia. Tuberculosis has been effectively ruled out at this point and bacterial pneumonia does not fit this clinical picture or any of the results. Asbestosis would cause parenchymal fibrosis and involves lower lobes. The bronchoscopy findings are inconsistent with asbestosis. Wegener's is on the differential as mentioned above but we have no evidence of renal disease and it is much rarer than Sarcoid in the African-American population.

---

65. Answer: D

The answer is restrictive ventilatory defect and marked decrease in diffusing capacity. Note that FVC and FEV_1 are reduced in parallel—this suggests a restrictive ventilatory defect. The marked decrease in diffusing capacity suggests loss of capillary surface area, which may be seen in pulmonary fibrosis, emphysema, or pulmonary vascular disease.

---

66. Answer: D

The answer is cavitary rheumatoid nodules. This man's major pulmonary findings were the cavitary rheumatoid nodules. Cancer and infection were excluded by histology and culture. Given the pattern of angiitis and granulomatosis (nodules), Wegener's granulomatosis (WG) could not be excluded histologically. The lack of upper respiratory and renal abnormalities and the presence of known rheumatoid arthritis in which similar histologic findings occur favored the diagnosis of rheumatoid angiitis and nodules.

67. Answer: C

This patient has had a pulmonary embolism. There is an increased risk of thromboembolic disease during pregnancy with possible contributing factors including:

- Decreased vasomotor tone due to increased prostaglandins
- Venous compression by the gravid uterus
- Hypercoagulability due to increased levels of coagulation factors I, II, VIII, IX, and X.
- Decreased plasma fibrinolytic activity.

This patient had her onset of pulmonary embolism approximately 1 week ago. Thrombolytic therapy is as effective if started in 6-14 days as compared to within 5 days of pulmonary embolism.

Her ECG is classic. The S1, Q3, T3 pattern is what is classically described but usually not seen. Echocardiogram is consistent with PE. With treatment and resolution her tricuspid regurgitation disappeared. Her right ventricle also returned to normal size as did her pulmonary artery systolic pressure.

68. Answer: B

The answer is fat embolism. Based on the findings of dyspnea, confusion, and petechiae (particularly neck, conjunctiva, and axilla [not described in this patient]) you can make the diagnosis of fat emboli in the face of a recent large bone fracture. Fat emboli can also occur after aggressive CPR and with sickle-cell bone occlusive crisis. Treatment is supportive; unless the patient has secondary ARDS, steroids have NOT proven of benefit. We don't give you a lot of lab values here and you shouldn't need them at this point. Again, the triad of dyspnea, confusion, and petechiae in the face of recent fracture…think of fat embolism!!

69. Answer: E

The correct answer is to admit to the hospital, place chest tube, and start intravenous ceftriaxone. He has an empyema by definition: He has organisms seen on gram stain! The organism is likely pneumococcus. Because he has an empyema you must place the chest tube as soon as possible; he will not get better without drainage of the pus. Intravenous antibiotics alone will not work. Waiting 24 hours or consulting a pulmonologist will not change the basic fact that he needs "draino"!!! If you chose to send this patient home you get 20 lashes with a wet noodle. Remember: organisms on gram stain of pleural fluid = NEEDS CHEST TUBE. Finally, the choice to add gentamicin for synergy is not correct. It is only useful for synergy for *Staphylococcus*, group B *Streptococcus*, *Listeria*, and *Enterococcus* infections.

70. Answer: A

The answer is *Staphylococcus aureus*. She has had recent influenza and this is the classic setting where Staphylococcal pneumonia will occur. *Streptococcus pneumoniae* is still very common in these patients also. Influenza virus is known both to increase respiratory colonization by *S. aureus* and to impair ciliary function (and therefore clearance of staphylococci).

71. Answer: E

The correct answer is to continue current therapy. Clinically she is doing well; you are weaning her off the vent; her physical examination is stable; her laboratory is stable (NEVER BASE ANTIBIOTIC THERAPY on a MINOR BUMP IN WBC). The sputum results are not unusual for a patient in the Intensive Care Unit; they will frequently become colonized with gram-negative organisms—particularly *Pseudomonas*. Never change therapy based on just a tracheal aspirate…you must have some other change in exam or laboratory that is significant for you to consider treating the organism found on a tracheal aspirate.

72. Answer: D

The answer is *Francisella tularensis*. You need to put together the following: He is from Arkansas—if you see this state think: Blastomycosis, Histoplasmosis, Ehrlichiosis and Tularemia (a mnemonic for those of you mnemonically-driven: BHET - Bill and Hilary Eat Toads in Arkansas). Secondly, he is a hunter in Arkansas: say the 4 organisms again! Third, he has a pneumonia that is unresponsive to ceftriaxone—think an unusual organism, which could be any of our 4 choices (BHET). Finally, they tell you that he is growing a gram-negative rod. Put Arkansas, pneumonia and gram-negative rod together and there is only one choice: tularemia, which is caused by *Francisella tularensis*.

73. Answer: A

Ok. If you didn't get the right answer here get on the floor and give me 50 push-ups. If you see the words pneumonia and San Joaquin Valley, go for coccidioidomycosis (by the way, do you know how difficult it is to spell and type coccidioidomycosis?? Try it. The spell checker at MedStudy is tired just from me using this dang word so many times in this one question.) Now read the question through because occasionally--very occasionally--they will throw in a simple Pneumococcal pneumonia on someone who lives in a weird part (Oops..sorry if you are from the San Joaquin Valley, I don't mean that you are "weird"—you know what I mean) of the country just to be sure you know that common things are common and rare things are rare. BUT, they will make it very clear they have something mundane like pneumococcal pneumonia: fever, a shaking chill, rusty sputum, etc….

74. Answer: A

The correct answer is *Chlamydia pneumoniae*. With the history of prior sore throat and now a febrile illness with documented pneumonia by chest x-ray, *Chlamydia pneumoniae* is the most likely. The stupid parrot is a red herring here as she had no signs of *C. psittaci* infection—look for a pneumonia with an extensive interstitial pattern that appears to be much worse than the physical exam would indicate. *C. trachomatis,* remember, causes genitourinary disease. *Staphylococcal aureus* would be seen after an influenza-like illness or if she were immunocompromised and she would be much sicker. Don't be thrown by the positive throat culture for this organism--it can be found frequently in asymptomatic people. *H. influenzae* should not cause pneumonia in her age group.

75. Answer: C

The answer is azithromycin 500 mg 2 po today, then 1 po q day x 4 days . She could have *Streptococcus pneumoniae, Mycoplasma pneumoniae,* or *Chlamydia pneumoniae*. Azithromycin and gatifloxacin are the only agents listed that are effective against all 3 organisms. The problem is that she is 17—note the ABIM will follow the FDA rules. You cannot give a quinolone to a child under the age of 18 except in special circumstances (anthrax, cystic fibrosis patients, etc.). The Beta-lactam antibiotics listed are great for pneumococcus but won't get the atypicals. In an adolescent with uncomplicated pneumonia, look for a macrolide or doxycycline as an acceptable choice.

76. Answer: D

The answer is to start INH 300 mg daily for 9 months. He is a recent converter. He has had a 10 mm increase in 1 year's time. By definition he should receive prophylaxis. His CXR is normal and he has no signs or symptoms of tuberculosis, therefore he does not need to be treated for active tuberculosis. 12 months of INH is no longer recommended for anyone, including HIV-infected patients! It is not reasonable to repeat the PPD in 2 weeks; he has a positive result and it will not change with repeated testing.

77. Answer: D

The answer is a PPD containing 5 TU of tuberculin without controls. The use of "control" testing is no longer recommended by the American Thoracic Society or the CDC for any patient routinely. Therefore, the use of controls should be discouraged. Even though she is severely immunocompromised, a standard PPD is still appropriate. NEVER, EVER pick the 250 TU on a test. There is no reason to use it so you can effectively mark out those answers when you see them listed on a test! The 2-step (or boosted) PPD has no place in routine practice; it is generally reserved for people who are repeatedly tested such as health-care workers.

78. Answer: D

The person who should NOT receive prophylaxis therapy is the patient with the PPD reading at 72 hours of 7 mm who is immunocompromised with leukemia on 5 mg/day of prednisone. According to the guidelines, the cut-off is 10 mm for this patient. All of the other patients require treatment; generally you would use INH for 9 months in each of these other patients. If this patient had been on 15 mg or more of daily prednisone then they would have met the criteria for therapy.

79. Answer: E

The answer is none needed unless clinical symptoms/problems develop. He is a healthy person without evidence of liver disorder. If he had during the initial evaluation evidence to suggest a liver disorder, then he should have baseline serum aspartate aminotransferase (AST) or serum alanine aminotransferase (ALT) and bilirubin drawn. Baseline testing is also indicated for patients with HIV infection, pregnant women, and women in the immediate postpartum period (within 3 months of delivery), persons with a history of chronic liver disease (hepatitis B or C, alcoholic hepatitis, or cirrhosis), persons who use alcohol regularly, and persons at risk for chronic liver disease. Baseline testing is NO LONGER routinely indicated in older persons (>35 y/o). But for patients with chronic conditions on medications that could cause problems, testing may be warranted. Guidelines do not say how often to do laboratory testing but probably q monthly is a good idea in those patients who require baseline screening.

Now clinical monitoring is indicated! This includes educating patients about signs and symptoms that might indicate a problem with the medication. These include any of the following: unexplained anorexia, nausea, vomiting, dark urine, icterus, rash, persistent paresthesias of the hand and feet, persistent fatigue, weakness or fever lasting 3 or more days, abdominal tenderness (especially right upper quadrant discomfort), easy bruising or bleeding, and arthralgia. Clinical monitoring begins at the first visit and should be done monthly.

80. Answer: C

The answer is ethambutol toxicity. Ethambutol is generally not hepatotoxic, but will cause problems with visual acuity, particularly color perceptions. The other agents are not associated with this problem.

81. Answer: D

The correct answer is lumbar puncture. She has cryptococcal lung disease and there is a high risk of dissemination to the central nervous system with this organism. You aren't really going to have to identify, say, a Histoplasma from a Cryptococcus, but you will need to know the more common organisms for an immunocompromised person to get. A person with lymphoma like this patient is at increased risk for cryptococcal infection, Coccidiodes infection, and aspergillus infection. If we had said she was from the San Joaquin Valley—then it is a no-brainer, right?? Aspergillus, remember, is branching. If they show you Cryptococcus they will likely show it to you with the nice capsule that you remember from 2nd year Microbiology.

82. Answer: C

The answer is to start enteral feeds as soon as possible. Enteral feeds are preferred over TPN because enteral feeds will maintain the intestinal epithelium and its natural defenses against bacteria. There is no reason to make this patient NPO.

83. Answer: C

The answer is nasal continuous positive airway pressure (CPAP). The continuous pressure "splints" the nasopharynx open at night. It is uncomfortable for many patients and some prefer the use of BiPAP instead, which allows for independent adjustment for inspiration and expiratory pressures. Sleeping supine and using hypnotics actually would worsen OSA. Sleeping under a fan would not have any effect. The type of television show shouldn't affect this either—although I know of no scientific study to prove this wrong.

84. Answer: D

The correct answer is squamous cell. Squamous cell more commonly involves the central/hilar area with local extension and is the most likely cancer to cavitate. Also, it is most commonly associated with hypercalcemia (large cell is next). Adenocarcinoma and large cell are usually peripheral. Bronchoalveolar carcinoma is just a subtype of adenocarcinoma. Squamous and small cell are usually central (remember the S-S sounds like Sentral). With small cell, cavitation NEVER occurs.

S S S

So if you put together central lesions, this leaves squamous and small cell; then put in cavitation and that only leaves squamous left—plus for an added bonus, squamous is the one most commonly to have hypercalcemia.

85. Answer: D

The answer is small cell carcinoma. Let's put this together. It is central--which means it is either Small Cell or Squamous Cell (Remember S-S-Sentral). Now, you presume from the information that the patient has SIADH—

that generally is associated with small cell. Therefore putting together central carcinoma with SIADH and you get small cell as the answer.
Adenocarcinoma, large cell, and bronchoalveolar (a type of adenocarcinoma) are usually peripheral.

---

86. Answer: E

The correct answer is after surgical resection, no further therapy is indicated. She has a very localized lesion to the lung. She does not have any nodal involvement and has no metastases. Also, she has a non-small cell type of cancer, so surgical resection should be sufficient. She does not need further therapy at this point.

---

87. Answer: A

The answer is *Coxiella burnetii*. For this case, the fact that he worked with animal placentas should make you think about *Coxiella burnetii*—remember if you see some type of animal "placenta" or birthing event then consider *Coxiella burnetii*—recent literature has had outbreaks with CATS—so be suspicious if Tabby is around delivering kittens and people are getting pneumonia. The other clue that this might be *Coxiella* is the marked hepatosplenomegaly. This is one of those "pneumonia with splenomegaly" organisms.

---

88. Answer: D

The correct answer is systemic corticosteroids. The key here is that she has Allergic Bronchopulmonary Aspergillosis (ABPA). The treatment for this is steroids and not anti-fungal agents. If you see something fungal that is branching it is likely aspergillus, especially if there is "right-angle" or 90-degree branching.

---

89. Answer: E

The answer is no further work-up is needed. Calcified nodules are benign. And in this patient, being that he is from Mississippi, histoplasmosis is a likely etiology. They do not require further work-up. If he had a "popcorn" calcified pattern then you would schedule a follow-up CXR over a period of 2 years to be sure it didn't get bigger; as this is likely a hamartoma. Solitary nodules WITHOUT calcifications are also watched for 2 years in low-risk patients (on the TEST)—in the real world we all know we work these things up and the answer is benign 99% of the time).

---

90. Answer: A

The correct answer is alveolar hypoventilation alone. The differential diagnosis of arterial hypoxemia includes all of the above plus decreased diffusion and high altitude (low FiO2). While this patient is at risk for aspiration pneumonia, pulmonary edema and other underlying pulmonary pathology, a quick calculation of the A-a gradient on room air reveals a normal A-a gradient. (150- (50+ 72/0.8) = A-a gradient of 10. The A-a gradient is increased in all causes of hypoxemia except hypoventilation and high altitude. We were not given any information that this patient was found on the summit in Aspen, therefore alveolar hypoventilation due to the presumed narcotic injection is the physiological mechanism for hypoxemia in this patient.

91. Answer: C

The correct answer is to transfuse 2 units packed red blood cells. This patient is still only partially resuscitated with evidence for both hemorrhagic shock and the hyperdynamic phase of SIRS (systemic inflammatory response syndrome). Most importantly is the continued acidosis, which is predominantly a metabolic acidosis and presumably a lactic acidosis indicating inadequate tissue perfusion. The best way to continue the resuscitation is to improve oxygen delivery (DO2) to the tissues and monitor the ABG and lactate level to assess improvement. Oxygen delivery is determined by cardiac output, hemoglobin, and oxygen saturation. In this case the CO is already high and the oxygen saturation with a PO2 of 85 is at least 90%. Increasing the PO2 will not provide much more hemoglobin saturation. Therefore the best way to improve oxygen delivery is to increase the hemoglobin through additional packed red cell transfusions. Increasing the minute ventilation to compensate for the metabolic acidosis will only mask the problem. Dobutamine will reduce the systemic vascular resistance even more, resulting in further hypotension. Dopamine will increase the blood pressure and cause further tachycardia with no improvement in oxygen delivery to the tissues.

92. Answer: E

The correct answer is bronchoprovocation (Methacholine challenge test). With a normal cardiovascular and pulmonary exam, the most likely cause of the episodic dyspnea in this patient under 40 years of age is asthma. As asthma is episodic and reversible airways obstruction, spirometry performed while the patient is asymptomatic may well be normal. The best test to prove asthma is the methacholine bronchoprovocation test which will reveal hyper-reactive airways – the hallmark of asthma. If the patient had rales on the exam and was older, the possibility of an interstitial lung disease would have to be entertained and an HRCT of the chest would be indicated. Remember:, 10% of patients with interstitial lung disease will have a normal chest x-ray at the time of presentation. If the patient gave a history of chest pain or syncope with exertion and physical exam revealed a right parasternal heave and an accentuated P2, then the diagnosis of pulmonary hypertension by echocardiography would be warranted. If an upper airway obstruction was suggested by the history or the patient was found to have stridor, a flow-volume loop would be a good screening test for upper airway obstruction. A normal ABG with a normal A-a gradient would make a diffusing capacity limitation unlikely.

93. Answer: E

The correct answer is no pulmonary function tests prior to surgery. Pre-operative PFTs and blood gasses are recommended for patients with underlying lung disease who are to undergo operative procedures that are in proximity to the diaphragm. An FEV1 less than 1 liter and arterial blood gasses revealing hypoxemia and/or respiratory acidosis would place the patient at a higher risk for postoperative pulmonary complications (prolonged mechanical ventilation, pneumonia, atelectasis). This patient requires no further testing as his asthma is stable and the procedure is not in proximity to the diaphragm.

94. Answer: D

The correct answer is inhaled corticosteroid, twice daily plus B-2 agonist as needed. This patient has asthma that would be characterized as Moderate-Persistent by the National Asthma Education and Prevention Program Guidelines. As such, she should be on daily medication with an inhaled corticosteroid and a short-acting inhaled B-2 agonist as needed for symptoms. The emphasis on utilizing anti-inflammatory therapies (inhaled corticosteroids) was a major focus on the NAEPP guidelines for any asthma patient characterized as mild-persistent or greater. This was to overcome the over-reliance on symptomatic relief with B-2 agonist inhalers and the rising number of asthma deaths (most clutching their B-agonist inhalers and on no steroids!). A B-2 agonist inhaler must be available for symptomatic relief with the understanding that more frequent use of the B-agonist inhaler indicates a need for stepped-up anti-inflammatory therapy (higher dose inhaled steroids, PO prednisone). Long-acting B-agonist inhalers may be helpful but cannot be used for immediate relief of symptoms in an acute exacerbation. This means your patient would need three inhalers – an inhaled corticosteroid as well as both long-acting and short-acting B-2 agonist inhalers. Sustained release theophylline may help with nocturnal symptoms but has no anti-inflammatory action. Inhaled cromolyn alone can take weeks to start working and is best used in atopic asthma in children.

95. Answer: A

The correct answer is nasal oxygen, 1-2 L/min with follow-up ABG in 20 minutes. Increase oxygen flow based on the ABG to a PO2 of 55-60 mmHg. The treatment imperative is to provide this patient with supplemental oxygen to achieve a hemoglobin saturation of 88-90%. This is to prevent further hypoxemia, which can cause cardiac arrhythmias and acute cor pulmonale. Oxygen supplementation may result in worsening respiratory acidosis. (HINT: NOT through reduction in respiratory drive – COPD patients are just like the rest of us – our chemiotaxic centers for the control of ventilation are CO2 sensitive, not O2 driven!) Worsening respiratory acidosis can only be detected by ABGs, not pulse oximetry. If providing supplemental FiO2 to achieve an oxygen saturation of 88-90% results in severe respiratory acidosis, then positive pressure ventilation via non-invasive positive pressure ventilation or conventional ventilation must be considered.

96. Answer: A

The correct answer is open-lung biopsy. Full PFTs would only provide confirmation of what you already expect – this patient has an interstitial lung disease with probable restricted lung volumes and a reduced diffusing capacity. You need to know what ILD the patient has and how to stage it in terms of activity to decide on treatment options. In a young man with no suspicion of sarcoid or an infectious etiology, you would proceed to open lung biopsy. Transbronchial biopsy could be entertained if we felt a strong suspicion for sarcoid or an infectious etiology. The yield on transbronchial biopsy is very good for these etiologies. However, in order to provide an adequate tissue sample for examination, an open lung biopsy (traditional or thorascopic) is required. In patients greater than 70 years of age, with no evidence of occupational, medication, or environmental exposure, this presentation would be classic for idiopathic pulmonary fibrosis and you could skip the open-lung biopsy. In these patients, an HRCT may provide a clue to the staging of the disease (ground-glass appearing airspace disease suggest active cellular component, not burnt out fibrosis).

97. Answer: D

The correct answer is delayed (Type IV, cell mediated) skin test reaction to *A. fumigatus*. All of the above are considered minor or major criteria for the diagnosis of ABPA except that there is no Type IV, cell mediated skin reaction. There are Type I and Type III (erythema and induration) skin test reactions. ABPA should be a consideration in any asthmatic who clinically worsens with repeated attacks despite adherence to therapy.

98. Answer: D

The correct answer is idiopathic bronchiolitis obliterans with organizing pneumonia (BOOP). While histologic confirmation is warranted, this is a classic presentation of BOOP. The flu-like illness that has not responded to antibiotics is a favorite of the ABIM. Histologic confirmation is needed because the patient will need a prolonged course (6-12 months) of corticosteroids and possible additional immunosuppressive agents. ABPA is unlikely as there is no prior history of asthma. Loeffler's is a self-limiting benign eosinophilic pneumonia that is asymptomatic. IPF or other interstitial lung diseases are in the differential, but the time course is a little short and we have no occupational, environmental, or medication history. Hypersensitivity pneumonitis is not suggested by the history, and frequently the patient would appear more ill and have basilar rales on auscultation.

---

99. Answer: B

The correct answer is echocardiogram. This is one of the ABIM's favorites. Look for the young woman with exertional dyspnea, chest pain, and has physical exam findings consistent with right heart strain. The next step in the work-up is an echocardiogram to document the existence of pulmonary hypertension and exclude significant mitral stenosis. After echocardiographic documentation of pulmonary hypertension, the work-up would proceed in the absence of any discernible parenchymal lung disease to V/Q scan to look for thromboembolic disease. A pulmonary angiogram would be helpful in evaluating any perfusion defects seen on V/Q. The role of right heart catheterization is further down the road when you are considering vasodilator therapy in the patient with primary pulmonary hypertension.

We do not suspect cardiac ischemia. Pulmonary function tests (particularly diffusion capacity) are helpful in assessing severity in documented cases of pulmonary hypertension, but have little use in the initial work-up of the patient unless you suspect secondary pulmonary hypertension from underlying COPD.

---

100. Answer: A

The correct answer is tuberculosis. This effusion is clearly exudative, hemorrhagic, and with a lymphocytic predominance. There were no mesothelial cells noted. Tuberculosis pleuritis is common in elderly patients and should be a leading consideration in this case. Confirmation via fluid AFB stain and culture and/or pleural biopsy with culture should be performed. The absence of parenchymal or nodal disease leads us away from suspecting parapneumonic, lymphoma, or bronchogenic carcinoma. The negative pleural cytology rules out malignant mesothelioma.

---

101. Answer: E

The correct answer is no testing – observe the patient. You are going to get a question on histo or blastomycosis. I like this question as it keeps with the ABIM's theme of doing nothing!

This patient has acute histoplasmosis from the neighborhood barn cleaning party. The neighborhood outbreak is not uncommon when there is land cleared or bulldozed. The key is that histoplasmosis is usually a self-limited disease for which we do not consider treatment unless there is evidence for progression to more disseminated disease. Accurate diagnosis relies on the history of exposure. Histoplasmin skin tests are useless, as many people will test positive after exposure without having the disease. Cultures are not very sensitive and may take weeks to grow. A positive culture from sputum or tissue is diagnostic, however. Serologic testing is not very sensitive and does not provide a timely diagnosis.

---

102. Answer: D

The correct answer is obtain prior chest x-rays for comparison. When a lung lesion is first identified in a patient it is imperative to determine whether the lesion is, in fact, new or old. If the lesion is old then you want to evaluate the stability of the lesion (no appreciable growth over 2 years.) Therefore, the first step is to obtain any old films. If there are no prior films, the next step is a CT scan of the chest with contrast to evaluate the presence of disease.

If this is demonstrated, then bronchoscopy is indicated to look for endobronchial involvement and rule out an infectious etiology for the lesion. If bronchoscopy is not helpful, there is some controversy whether it is best to perform transthoracic needle biopsy or just go to surgical removal of the lesion. The decision involves whether your patient would tolerate a thoracotomy and whether a non-diagnostic transthoracic needle biopsy (atypia, inflammatory Schmutz) would just mandate a thoracotomy anyway.

103. Answer: B

The correct answer is polysomnography with trial of nasal continuous positive airway pressure (CPAP). The probability of this patient having serious obstructive sleep apnea is high. He is a threat to himself, the community, and his marriage. There is little time to waste. Therefore a "split-study" polysomnography should be ordered such that the technician performing the study can analyze the results during the first part of the study and institute a trial of nasal CPAP if the preliminary result is unequivocally positive for serious obstructive sleep apnea (greater than 15 significant apnea/hypopnea events per hour). In this way a patient can be started on nocturnal nasal CPAP as soon as possible. While weight loss, alcohol avoidance, and exercise are important instructions, it is unlikely that these measures alone will work in the short term in this patient. Uvulopalatopharyngoplasty is an alternative treatment for obstructive sleep apnea, but the results to date are inferior to CPAP. Amphetamines and tricyclic antidepressants are used to treat narcolepsy.

104. Answer: B

The correct answer is assist/control mode, Rate 12/min, Tidal Volume 700cc, Peak flow 80 L/min. Many of you are surprised that the ABIM expects you to have much knowledge about mechanical ventilation. I know, that's what pulmonologists are for... BUT the ABIM also recognizes that internists do take care of critically ill patients without the availability of subspecialists and that patients are getting hurt. Therefore this type of question is fair game.

We all recognize that the hemodynamic demise in this patient was from dynamic hyperinflation and the creation of auto-PEEP. (I painstakingly gave you enough information to exclude a tension pneumothorax.) Just think of air trapping and breath "stacking." This patient's underlying problem is expiratory airflow obstruction. So what did the ED doctor do? In an effort to immediately reverse the acute hypercapnic respiratory failure, he hyperventilated the patient and provided a large tidal volume at a low peak flow rate.* (Peak flow determines how fast the gas is delivered for each breath – a higher peak flow results in the breath being delivered quickly (short inspiratory time), allowing for a longer expiratory phase.) This patient could not possibly have had enough time to empty his lungs with each breath. Ultimately he builds up such a large pressure in his chest (auto-PEEP) that blood flow return is compromised and hypotension ensues. In removing the patient from mechanical ventilation, you allowed the trapped gas to be released and hemodynamic stability returned. While tempting to leave the patient on a T-Bar without any positive pressure, I assure you that he will quickly tire and have a respiratory arrest.

Therefore, you return the patient to mechanical ventilation (Assist/control mode is as good as any) with the understanding that you want a tidal volume of 5-10 ml/kg, a high peak flow rate, and a lower respiratory rate (8-14). Even without sophisticated monitoring you should be able to see that you are not trapping air by auscultating the lungs through a few respiratory cycles and see that the patient has finished his expiration phase before the next breath by the ventilator is delivered. Recognize that this method of ventilating the patient may well not fully correct his respiratory acidosis. That's ok, a moderate amount of respiratory acidosis is well tolerated (permissive hypercapnia), so aim to get a pH > 7.20 as your initial goal and let the bronchodilators, steroids etc. start to work.

105. Answer: A

The correct answer is high cardiac output, low systemic vascular resistance, and low wedge pressure. The ABIM has not allowed internists to leave the critical care stuff to the intensivists. Utilizing a Swan-Ganz catheter to generate a hemodynamic profile of shock such as above is a reasonable question for the exam. They may even throw in more data such as pulmonary artery pressure, mixed venous oxygen saturation and even left ventricular stroke volume to foul you up. Stick to the parameters above and you should be able to narrow down the answer sufficiently.
Remember the hallmark of early, "warm" sepsis is a hyperdynamic heart (increased cardiac output) coupled with a very low systemic vascular resistance. Typically the patient in early septic shock is volume depleted and "third spacing" a considerable amount of the fluids given for resuscitation due to the low systemic vascular resistance. In all the other entities above, the systemic vascular resistance is high as it is the only thing holding the blood pressure together!

Hypovolemic shock, whether hemorrhagic or intravascular volume depletion is characterized by a low wedge pressure, a reduced cardiac output, and a high SVR.
Cardiogenic shock is defined by a low cardiac output, high-filling pressures (think CHF), and a high SVR.
Obstructive shock is typified by a massive PE or a tension pneumothorax. There is reduced cardiac filling, reduced cardiac output, and a high SVR. In pericardial tamponade the filling pressures will be normal as a reduced volume is acted on by a decreased compliance of the ventricular wall.

106. Answer: A

The correct answer is methylene blue. This patient presents with hypotension and cyanosis. He was at a party when the symptoms started. This presentation is suggestive of nitrite abuse. He most likely used amyl nitrite ("poppers") at the party. The nitrite induces methemoglobinemia, which causes the cyanosis unresponsive to oxygen administration. Administration of methylene blue will reduce ferric iron to its ferrous state, resolving the methemoglobinemia.

107. Answer: C

The correct answer is quantitative ventilation scan. The only cure for lung cancer is a surgical resection. As such, we strive to make any patient a surgical candidate. This patient's pre-op PFTs show an FEV1 less than 2.0 liters – the traditional cutoff for surgical candidates. Smoking cessation, inhaled steroids, and further intervention from a pulmonologist may improve his FEV1, but at the risk of delaying the curative procedure. Therefore, as there are asymmetrical bullae on the CT scan, it is likely that the ventilation scan will show less ventilation to the right lung and a quantitative assessment would allow even a right pneumonectomy.

108. Answer: B

The correct answer is order an EKG and echocardiogram to evaluate for cor pulmonale. As a consultant I am often faced with this dilemma. HCFA and the Office of Inspector General will not tolerate fraud! For insurance to cover this man's home oxygen you would need to demonstrate evidence of cor pulmonale in addition to his blood gas results. His Hct does not qualify him on the basis of erythrocytosis.

109. Answer: B

The correct answer is bilateral peripheral infiltrates. This presentation of a 40-year-old woman with a history of asthma is classic for chronic eosinophilic pneumonia. The CXR is classically referred to as the "photographic negative" of pulmonary edema. ABPA would be suggested by a history of coughing brownish sputum and the subsequent mucous plugging that can lead to segmental atelectasis on chest x-ray. There is always a possibility of pulmonary tuberculosis, but the eosinophilia would not be a hallmark.

---

110. Answer: D

The correct answer is high-resolution CT of the chest. Nearly 10% of patients presenting with interstitial lung disease will have a normal CXR. High-resolution chest CT is the test of choice to evaluate for the presence of an interstitial lung disease. HRCT will be helpful diagnostically in assessing the distribution of the disease as well as providing guidance for a possible lung biopsy. In addition, HRCT may provide a clue to the staging of the disease (ground-glass appearing airspace disease suggests an active cellular component vs. burnt out fibrosis).

Full PFTs would only provide confirmation of what you already expect – this patient has an interstitial lung disease with probably restricted lung volumes and a reduced diffusing capacity. Flexible bronchoscopy with transbronchial biopsy could be entertained if we felt a strong suspicion for sarcoid or an infectious etiology. The yield on transbronchial biopsy is very good for these etiologies. However, in order to provide an adequate tissue sample for examination in most ILDs, an open lung biopsy (traditional or thorascopic) is required.

---

111. Answer: D

The answer is decrease in systolic BP > 15 mm Hg. Other things that should make you stop the test quickly are: ST segment depression greater than 2 mm; development of ventricular tachycardias; development of chest pain, shortness of breath, or lightheadedness. Remember that a positive test is indicated by finding ST depression of >1 mm that lasts longer than 0.08 seconds. His prior probability of heart disease is very high based on his symptoms and family history, so a positive test in this patient is likely a true positive.

---

112. Answer: B

The answer is RV infarction with secondary failure; administer normal saline. In this setting of a recent acute inferior MI and new recurrence of severe chest pain, you must be worried about RV infarction with secondary failure. The RV has decompensated and is unable to fill the left side. Treatment is to give FLUIDS until the blood pressure returns to normal. Think of this in a hypotensive patient with inferior MI!!

With pericardial tamponade you would get equal pressures in all 4 chambers.

For biventricular failure, you would expect low cardiac output, PCWP to be high, and RA pressure is high. Treatment listed is correct.

With mitral stenosis with secondary RV failure, you would see elevated RA pressure, elevated PA press, and elevated PCWP.

In pulmonary hypertension, you would see that the RA pressure is elevated and the PA diastolic pressure is markedly higher than the PCWP.

113. Answer: D

The answer is atrial fibrillation. This patient had acute onset of symptoms. As it turns out, his relatives Quince and Quatro had protein C deficiency. And guess what? So does this guy. His atrial fibrillation was from a big pulmonary embolism.

114. Answer: E

The correct answer is lidocaine. The most appropriate management of cardiac arrest induced by ventricular tachycardia (which is what the rhythm strip shows) is administering an initial 200-joule defibrillation. Additional shocks at higher energies up to a maximum of 360 joules should be attempted if the initial shock is ineffective in reverting the ventricular tachycardia. However, whether the initial defibrillation worked or not, lidocaine should be administered as a 1mg/kg bolus.

115. Answer: D

The correct answer is to insert a permanent cardiac pacemaker. What the ECG is describing is the sudden failure of atrial ventricular conduction without a preceding change in the PR interval. Ok now before I tell you, think a minute. By definition, what does Mr. Burns have?? That's correct, Mobitz type II second-degree AV block. This is BAD. It usually means significant disease of the conducting system. It is also an unstable thing to have and frequently will progress to complete heart block. Therefore, the only correct solution is to put in a permanent pacemaker in anticipation that he will continue to have worsening of his conduction abnormalities.

116. Answer: A

The correct answer to this question is right heart failure. Ankle edema does not equal heart failure!!!!!!!!!!!!!!!!!!!!!!!!! Look at her physical examination: she has no jugular venous distention—it is very, very unlikely for her to have heart failure with normal jugular pressures. All of the other items listed should be considered before you even think about right heart failure.

117. Answer: B

The correct answer is parenteral penicillin and aspirin. This patient has acute rheumatic fever. Remember, he needs two of the following major manifestations: carditis, migratory polyarthritis, chorea, erythema marginatum, and subcutaneous nodules. He has three of the five major criteria. Additionally, he has fever and evidence of recent group A Streptococcus infection with the positive ASO titer. Even if *Streptococcus pyogenes* cannot be isolated, you still treat them with a therapeutic course of 1.2 million units of IM penicillin as one dose or oral penicillin for 10 days. Most authorities recommend the IM injection in the setting of acute rheumatic fever. He would then go on prophylactic Penicillin q month to prevent recurrent attacks. Steroids are not indicated for treatment of the arthritis. The arthritis will usually respond quite well to aspirin. However, many believe that there is a role for steroids in patients with severe carditis accompanied by congestive heart failure. However, neither salicylates nor glucocorticoids influence the future development of valvular heart disease. In adults, prednisone can be started in doses as high as 30 mg four times daily in especially severe cases, and as the patient improves, salicylates can be added during the tapering of the steroid dose; this may require 4 to 6 weeks.

118. Answer: C

The answer is decrease of the murmur with handgrip. His echocardiogram showing evidence of a disproportionately thickened ventricular septum and systolic anterior motion of the mitral valve strongly suggests hypertrophic cardiomyopathy, also known as idiopathic hypertrophic subaortic stenosis (IHSS). The harsh systolic murmur that he has should not radiate to the carotids with this condition. Additionally, the murmur will decrease when he applies a handgrip—this will increase ventricular volume due to isometric exercise. The carotid upstroke is brisk and frequently is bifid. His congestive failure is likely occurring because of the reduced ventricular compliance despite NORMAL left ventricular systolic function. Mitral regurgitation is much more likely than is mitral stenosis.

119. Answer: C

The correct answer to this question is diffuse T-wave inversion with ST-segment elevation. Don't you just HATE these "LEAST" and "NOT" kinds of questions!!

Another way to think of this question: Which of these CAN or IS LIKELY to occur in pericarditis? Then pick the one that is left that DOES NOT fit—kind of a reverse psychology for yourself on the questions if you get confused. Look for what DOES do it and then see what is left as the EXCEPT.

Many of you probably went for the "no rub" answer. However, remember that a rub is actually not that common. So if we read the question as "Which of the following findings CAN occur in acute pericarditis?" then the finding of "NO RUB" is certainly a possibility. NOW, if the rub is there, it is diagnostic; if not, then it really doesn't help you rule out the diagnosis. With a pericarditis you would expect to see frequent atrial premature beats. Also, PR-segment depression, especially in Lead II, would help you here. CPK's will rise with pericarditis frequently and in fact can be 2-3 times normal; but they are TRANSIENTLY elevated. The finding of diffuse T-wave inversion with ST-segment elevation means the poor guy had an MI, not pericarditis. It would LEAST support the diagnosis of acute pericarditis.

120. Answer: A

The correct answer is infection transmitted by a bite from a tick. His picture is consistent with manifestations of Lyme disease, which is transmitted by the bite of an *Ixodes scapularis* (formerly *I. dammini*). Lyme disease is due to *Borrelia burgdorferi*. His exposure occurred while he was "moonlighting" off of Long Island, which is a high-risk area for Lyme disease. Lyme carditis is most often manifested by AV nodal conduction disturbances, anywhere from 1st through 3rd degree heart block. Treatment consists of a 3rd generation cephalosporin or high-dose parenteral penicillin therapy. IT will resolve usually with treatment.

Cocaine can cause myocardial ischemia and infarction, but we have no evidence on ECG that this has occurred and his symptoms have been prolonged now for a while, so the ECG should have some evidence of damage at this point. HIV carditis would not present this way. And a coronary artery embolus would not present in this fashion either over several days.

121. Answer: B

The correct answer is PVCs such as these (even this mild) can cause symptoms. Palpitations are the most common symptoms that people will perceive from them. Symptoms can also occur if the stroke volume is decreased by decreasing overall ventricular filling. PVCs are common and occur in nearly 60% of men who undergo Holter monitoring. In patients who have known coronary artery disease, the frequency and nature of the PVCs do matter; for example >10/hour is associated with increased mortality. PVCs increase in frequency with aging not decrease.

122. Answer: B

The correct answer is placement of a temporary pacing wire and stop her diltiazem and atenolol. Of course, you might want to kill yourself too after going through that long, dragged out Review of systems!! Stool glowing in the dark? Maybe we should call "The X-Files"?? (Plus, you know Medicare is only going to reimburse you $20 for this consult anyway…) Ok back to the answer. She has significant symptomatic bradycardia with spells of sinus arrest. This is most likely due to her medications, particularly the beta-blocker. Elderly patients can be particularly at risk for AV nodal blockade from beta-blockers and diltiazem, especially when used in combination. Thus, we could probably temporarily pace Ms. Perkins and then see if the bradycardia resolves off of the medications. She is symptomatic and has significant pauses so just stopping the medication alone would not be correct; a temporary pacer is needed at this point. Using atropine would not be effective for prolonged periods of time if this were drug induced; plus it is likely to cause her more harm.

123. Answer: E

The correct answer is hypertrophic cardiomyopathy (idiopathic hypertropic subaortic stenosis). He has all of the classic findings of hypertropic cardiomyopathy. He has a harsh systolic murmur without radiation to the neck. The murmur is due to the intracavitary obstruction in the left ventricle. The murmur increases with Valsalva or any other maneuver that will decrease left ventricular size, which will increase the outflow obstruction and the intensity of the murmur. Conversely, maneuvers that increase left ventricular blood volume (squatting and passive leg raising) will "move" the muscular obstruction protruding into the outflow track away from the opposite wall, decreasing the obstruction and the murmur. The brisk carotid upstroke is also part of this condition. Additionally the history was helpful; the death of his older brother suggests the "familial" form of this disease.

124. Answer: B

The correct answer is echocardiogram. This patient has hypertrophic cardiomyopathy (idiopathic hypertropic subaortic stenosis). All aspects of his physical examination correlate with this diagnosis: the harsh systolic murmur, the murmur increasing with standing and decreasing with squatting. The murmur does not radiate to the neck. The history of his brother dying of "sudden" death supports the familial form of this disease. An echocardiogram will show you the disproportionately thickened ventricular septum and systolic anterior motion of the mitral valve. A treadmill stress test will need to be done BUT you need nuclear images. Also, a Holter monitor is done to look for non-sustained episodes of V-tach. The ECG will be non-specific and won't make the diagnosis for you. It may show Q waves in the inferior to lateral leads (from the hypertrophied septum) and have a normal to increased voltage (depending on the degree of LVH). If the voltage is low, consider an infiltrative cardiomyopathy such as amyloid heart disease.

125. Answer: A

The answer is thrombolytics for treatment of an acute MI. This patient has acute pericarditis by his symptoms and physical examination. It is very unlikely that this healthy young man has had an MI. Diffuse concave-up ST elevation is seen with pericarditis as opposed to localized concave-down ST elevation seen in an acute MI.

Everything else listed you would do for symptomatic relief. Admission is warranted to follow his course and look for common etiologies, although it is likely that this will be idiopathic after his viral infection.

126. Answer: A

The correct answer is bicuspid aortic valve. 70% of people with coarctation will also have a bicuspid aortic valve. Usually signs such as murmurs, etc. don't occur until later in life in the mid-30s. None of the other conditions are commonly associated with coarctation. You probably thought I was going to ask you about her congenital condition—but this is a cardiology question, silly. You are right though – she does have Turner's syndrome. Note also that aneurysms of the circle of Willis occur with coarctation also.

127. Answer: C

The correct answer is transposition of the great vessels. Cyanosis is usually noted in the first day of life and progresses rapidly as the ductus arteriosus closes. Remember with this, the aorta comes off the right ventricle and the pulmonary artery from the left. Tetralogy of Fallot is the more common, but it won't show up until later in childhood. A trick question—how evil of me. But the boards want you to *think* on the exam also. Think about the anatomy—a baby is born with transposition—he/she will be cyanotic very quickly. With tetralogy the cyanosis won't occur for a while until the right ventricular outflow obstruction is progressive, usually not for the first few months of life. Later the kids get what is known as "tet" spells. These spells are hypoxic events and the child becomes restless and agitated and may cry inconsolably. Frequently children learn early on to "squat" and that helps increase systemic venous return resulting in more blood being made available to the pulmonary artery and increases systemic resistance, driving more venous blood into the lungs. Total anomalous pulmonary venous return is when there is a failure of incorporation of the common pulmonary vein into the posterior wall of the left atrium; this will cause severe cyanosis in the newborn period but is rarer than transposition. Tricuspid atresia will not usually cause cyanosis until around a year of age due to the presence of a VSD with this abnormality. VSD will not cause a cyanotic disease usually.

128. Answer: C

The correct answer is large VSD, right ventricular outflow tract obstruction, overriding aorta, RVH. This is just a simple memorization thing. It has appeared on past tests, so just memorize it. A mnemonic device that helps me is: "VROARV,"; where V stands for VSD, RO stands for right ventricular outflow obstruction, OA for overriding aorta, and RV for RVH. It may or may not help you—my brain is weird sometimes how it works. For some reason tetralogy of Fallot is one of those favorite questions over time. If you are Med/Peds you've got an added bonus here to help you with the Peds boards.

129. Answer: D

The correct answer is to do a Holter study. She likely is having an arrhythmia (such as SVT) from her caffeine intake. The best test would be to monitor on a Holter and then see what arrhythmia is occurring. The other tests are not indicated at this time.

130. Answer: D

The answer is dobutamine stress echo. He is diabetic and has some symptoms suggestive of coronary artery disease. He cannot perform a routine stress test due to his arthritis. An electrophysiologic study is not going to tell us anything. This could be an ulcer, but the pressing issue is whether or not he has coronary artery disease. Proceeding to left heart catheterization is invasive and not necessary at this point. The dobutamine stress echo should be helpful in determining if he has significant coronary disease—if so, then a left heart cath would be indicated.

131. Answer: C

The correct answer for this question is starting nitroprusside or nitroglycerin IV for afterload reduction. That would be the ONE thing here you would NOT want to do. His blood pressure is already low and he is in cardiogenic shock. You do not want afterload reduction—this will make his hypotension acutely worse. All of the other choices are appropriate depending on the hospital setting you are in. Obviously, if a cath lab was not available then the use of inotropic agents and placement of a Swan-Ganz would be best.

132. Answer: C

The correct answer is to add an ACE inhibitor. Adding the ACE inhibitor will increase cardiac output and decrease LV filling pressure due to the vasodilatory effect. ACE inhibitors block formation of angiotensin II, causing an increase in renin (from decreased negative feedback). They also have been shown to prolong survival. Increasing the digoxin dose would not be a good idea based on his current digoxin level, as well as current response to therapy. There is no need to go to a loop diuretic at this point as the hydrochlorothiazide is working well. A calcium channel blocker would not be effective and could be harmful. A calcium channel blocker would be effective if he had diastolic dysfunction.

133. Answer: D

The correct answer is to schedule surgery in 3 months, if clinically unchanged. In the majority of cardiac patients having noncardiac surgery, the highest potential risk is from coronary artery disease. In this patient with a history of recent MI, the incidence of reinfarction during a major noncardiac surgery averages approximately 6%. The risk however is inversely proportional to the time since the MI. For example, within the first 3 months the risk is 37%; after 6 months it falls to 4-5%. In this patient it would be better to wait another 3 months before doing this elective surgery. Additionally, he is having exercise-testing daily with his skating to work for 3 miles and his lawn mowing on the weekend. Studies have shown that an exercise capacity of 5-6 METs indicates that cardiac risk during noncardiac surgery is low. Mowing the lawn easily reaches this threshold; therefore, formal testing is not indicated and is just an added expense.

134. Answer: C

The correct answer is to decrease the propranolol dose. Be aware that patients of Asian descent may have an increased sensitivity to the effects of beta-blockers. The easiest thing is to decrease the dosing interval to twice a day and see if that works. The other tests are not indicated. Remember, he is asymptomatic so insertion of a temporary pacemaker is not indicated at this point.

135. Answer: D

The correct answer is vascular surgery consultation for aneurysm repair. She has an infrarenal abdominal aortic aneurysm that has surpassed the threshold level of 5 cm. Below 5 cm, these aneurysms are low risk for rupture. However, now that she has been found to have a 5.4 cm aneurysm, the best choice is to proceed with surgery.

136. Answer: B

The correct answer is to notify your cardiovascular surgeon to come right away and evaluate her for emergent mitral valve replacement. She has likely had a papillary muscle rupture and developed acute mitral insufficiency. The murmur is classically a holosystolic murmur at the APEX as opposed to being located at the left sternal border with acute ventricular septal defects. Cardiocentesis is not indicated, as she has no evidence indicating tamponade, which you would see with a left ventricular free wall rupture. The lack of syncope also points more toward ruptured papillary muscle instead of ventricular septum rupture or left ventricular free wall rupture.

137. Answer: D

The correct answer is systolic ejection click and murmur. This would indicate significant risk for endocarditis. The other items are low risk and do not require prophylaxis.

138. Answer: C

The correct answer is hypertrophic cardiomyopathy. All of the other choices do not require prophylaxis. You would think that having a pacer with electrodes going directly into the heart would, but there is no increased risk. The systolic click alone does not warrant prophylaxis either; a murmur also is required.

139. Answer: B

The correct answer is initial placement of orthodontic bands. Evidently this is enough manipulation of the gums to produce enough trauma where prophylaxis is indicated. All of the other items listed do not require prophylaxis. It is comforting to know that every time people go in for their orthodontic "adjustment," that prophylaxis is not indicated.

140. Answer: D

The correct answer is No prosthetic joints do not require prophylaxis for routine dental visits. There is some controversy about the use of prophylaxis for prolonged surgery or surgery involving infected areas—then some authorities do recommend prophylaxis. But for routine dental procedures no prophylaxis is indicated. I made up the porcine hip replacement—wouldn't that be funny though? Let's say for the sake of giving you another freebee question here: what if she was having prolonged surgery of an infected area of her mouth? What antibiotic would you use that is listed above?? The answer then would be clindamycin. Remember, she has anaphylaxis to penicillin—you certainly would not use amoxicillin and you would be a little leery of using a cephalosporin too.

141. Answer: A

The correct answer is ampicillin 2 grams IM or IV plus gentamicin 1.5 mg/kg. He is at HIGH risk because of his prosthetic valve—other conditions placing you at high risk include previous endocarditis and those with surgically constructed systemic-pulmonary shunts or conduits. Patients at high risk like Crisp here need combination ampicillin and gentamicin for prophylaxis of genitourinary and gastrointestinal procedures. The choice of vancomycin with gentamicin would be appropriate if he were penicillin-allergic. Amoxicillin would be appropriate if he was a "moderate" risk patient, say, with hypertrophic cardiomyopathy or previous cardiac rheumatic fever. Vancomycin alone would be appropriate if he was of "moderate" risk and penicillin-allergic. The ampicillin/clindamycin combo would not be used for any prophylaxis-type therapy.

---

142. Answer: A

The correct answer is hypertrophic obstructive cardiomyopathy (HOCM or IHSS). The combination of...

1) "spike and dome" carotid pulse contour
2) similar apex cardiogram
3) holosystolic murmur
4) murmur augmentation by standing and ...
5) murmur augmentation by Valsalva strain
6) the Brockenbrough phenomenon
7) sudden death (resuscitated)

makes the diagnosis of hypertrophic (obstructive) cardiomyopathy inescapable here. The pure form of this disease is now known to be an autosomal dominant transmission, thus explaining the importance of investigating other members of the kindred, particularly in the type of scenario described. This entity is one of the several diagnoses that is customarily first considered when there is an acute event in an elite athlete, other entities worth consideration in this regard being WPW, Marfan physiology, anomalous coronary disease, and long QT_c syndrome.

Appropriate associations with the other entities mentioned might include:

Myxomatous mitral valve prolapse [MVP]: mid-systolic click
Ostium secundum atrial septal defect [ASD]: fixed splitting of S_{II}
Ostium primum atrioventricular septal defect [AVSD]: RBBB / LAHB
Acquired (muscular) ventricular septal defect [VSD]: myocardial infarction
Wolff-Parkinson-White syndrome [WPW]: delta waves
Congenital long QT syndrome (Romano-Ward): $QT_c > 0.43$-0.44

---

143. Answer: D

The correct answer is thyroid glands. This is the autosomal dominant kindred of Multiple Endocrine Neoplasia (MEN) syndrome, type II-b or III, with the characteristic combination of pheochromocytoma, medullary thyroid carcinoma, and diffuse gastrointestinal ganglioneuromatoses (as manifest grossly at the bedside by the tongue nodules). Medullary thyroid carcinoma (MTC) originates in the thyroid parafollicular C cells, those responsible for the secretion of thyrocalcitonin. It may be either sporadic or familial. Familial forms can be isolated or an expression of MEN kindred. Mutations of the RET proto-oncogene have been identified in the germline DNA of patients with familial MTC syndromes. Genetic testing can identify patients affected by MEN and familial MTC, allowing early diagnosis and possible cure. Total preventive thyroidectomy has been recommended in all carriers of RET genetic defects, even in families at risk with mutations of the 618 or 620 codon, because the penetrance of FMTC approaches 100%, and a 100% accordance between presence of the disease and gene carrier status is reported. This procedure would therefore represent the only possibility of achieving a 100% cure in subjects affected by familial medullary thyroid carcinoma.

The primary patient's pheochromocytoma is obvious and warrants careful pre-operative treatment prior to surgical removal. The historic role of phentolamine (as the Regitine® test) is worth mentioning, although diagnosis now depends on other methodologies. Phentolamine remains an effective treatment modality in the acute setting. Obeying the Law of Nines, approximately 90% of pheochromocytoma patients secrete predominantly norepinephrine. For the less common patient with epinephrine predominance, the use of phentolamine could result in abrupt hypotension as a result of the classical "pharmacologic reversal" phenomenon (wherein epinephrine is converted from a pressor to a depressor via blockade of the vasoconstrictive receptors and leaving the receptors "unopposed.")

---

144. Answer: A

The correct answer is mural thrombus formation on a ruptured or eroded atherosclerotic plaque. During the past 15 years, we have learned an enormous amount about the pathogenesis and treatment of unstable angina. In most cases of unstable rest angina, the pathogenesis is a mural thrombus formation on a ruptured or eroded atherosclerotic plaque. All of the other factors are legitimate entities, and could even be operative in this particular patient, the key to a correct answer in the MOST LIKELY concept, rather than attempting to focus on lesser issues.

---

145. Answer: C

The correct answer is urgent revascularization ("direct angioplasty"). The prognosis for the patient with cardiogenic shock in the setting of myocardial infarction is limited and is a function of the amount of lost myocardium. The threshold value is usually stated to be 40%; losses above that amount generally are those that account for shock. The patient with acute papillary muscle disruption or perforation of the interventricular septum represents special, uniquely surgical challenges. The patient described here was seen as nearly hopeless until the observation that some may improve dramatically given a successful catheter revascularization approach. Hence, the proper answer here may be re-phrased as the following: "The one approach that appears to have some promise is the use of acute interventional revascularization measures in the catheterization laboratory."

---

146. Answer: B

The correct answer is Atenolol. A patient like this with both hypertension and ischemic heart disease really does warrant the use of a beta-adrenolytic agent so that the "cardio-protective" properties of this drug family may be employed. In a patient with both obstructive pulmonary disease and peripheral vascular disease with claudication, this would be the perfect scenario for the preferential use of the selective agent such as atenolol (or metoprolol, etc.); use of propranolol in this setting would likely add a bronchospastic component such that the patient would almost become "asthmatic." Importantly, the use of beta-blockers of any kind is generally avoided in asthmatic patients, noting that the selectivity attributed to some members of the family is relative, not absolute, and considerably dose-dependent.

The appearance of the HOPE trail may change our views of "cardio-protection;" this is the first inference that the angiotensin-converting enzymes (ACE) inhibitors may have the same type of property, which has been ascribed to the beta-blockers. From a test-taker point of view, the choice of atenolol herein is simply the better choice than enalapril or losartan, although this may surely change in future years. Had the patient here described been a diabetic patient, the selection of the ACE inhibitor (enalapril) would have been the preferred answer.

---

147. Answer: A

The correct answer is classic polyarteritis nodosa (PAN). Visceral angiography may be necessary to establish this diagnosis. Biopsy of skin, kidney, or other tissues should demonstrate the typical fibrinoid necrosis. The nomenclature herein is consistent with that suggested by the Chapel Hill classification. Although often suggested otherwise in various sources, the association of the ANCA antibodies is not with this entity but with the following:

p-ANCA
1) microscopic polyarteritis (MPA)--involvement of venules, capillaries, arterioles
2) Churg-Strauss --eosinophilia

c-ANCA
3) Wegener's granulomatosis--upper respiratory involvement (sinuses)

Proper associations with the other entities mentioned include:
Kawasaki's disease--infantile coronary artery aneurysms
Takayasu's disease--aortic arch involvement in an Asian
Familial Mediterranean Fever—Sephardic Jewish renal amyloidosis

Classical PAN affecting medium-sized arteries is usually not associated with ANCA markers at all. If an antibody association is present, there may be evidence for hepatitis response in some patients.

---

148. Answer: C

The correct answer is tricuspid regurgitation. The patients of this nature are so familiar in some geographic settings that the diagnosis is nearly routine. The characteristic features of tricuspid regurgitation accompanied by septic pulmonary emboli and evidence of parenteral drug usage predict that *Staphylococcus aureus* will be isolated as the causative agent in the majority of cases. Some of these patients have even had their tricuspid valves removed rather than attempting to implant a prosthetic device in a patient who could return to bacteremia-associated behaviors (via relapse). This is something that can be done if the patient has no additional heart disease. An alternative to this approach might include a plastic repair of the native valve, a so-called "vegetectomy."

---

149. Answer: A

The correct answer is a calcium antagonist given intravenously [IV} cannot be selected safely as the initial treatment. While absolute statements are seldom possible in medicine, one in which you may be confident, is the following:

"Calcium antagonism is NEVER the treatment for a patient with wide-complex tachycardia in the emergency setting."

If the diagnosis were actually traditional ventricular tachycardia, the calcium antagonist would have no primary efficacy and would simply add the adverse effect of negative inotropicity. If the diagnosis were antidromic conduction of a supraventricular tachycardia in the setting of pre-excitation physiology, the calcium antagonist would retard conduction at the atrioventricular (AV) junction and thereby enhance anomalous antegrade conduction.

The majority of patients who present with ventricular tachycardia have underlying structural heart disease. However, there has been increasing appreciation of the existence of multiple forms of idiopathic ventricular tachycardia with distinct features and unique mechanisms. The most common form of idiopathic ventricular tachycardia originates from the right ventricular outflow tract, which is characterized by sensitivity to adenosine, and appears to be due to cyclic AMP-mediated triggered activity. Other forms of idiopathic ventricular tachycardia include intrafascicular left ventricular tachycardia due to reentry, which is sensitive to verapamil, and automatic, propranolol-sensitive ventricular tachycardia. Although the mechanism of verapamil-sensitive idiopathic left ventricular tachycardia (ILVT) is usually reentry, the actual reentrant circuit is not clearly understood. This latter entity would be the sole exception to the general rule stated above, one that would not apply directly to the acute scenario as described.

---

150. Answer: B

The correct answer is they must be aware of the risk of sudden death. Unfortunately, this is very much the truth, and indeed, most boys with classical Duchenne's muscular dystrophy will not live past 20 years. It is precisely for this reason that there are fundamentally no girls with the disease, despite the predictions of the Punnett Square; there are (literally) no fathers! Whereas the cause of death in many Duchenne boys will be the relentless chronic progression of cardiopulmonary disease, there is an important component of sudden death relating to the arrhythmias and conduction system disease accompanying their characteristic cardiomyopathy. The EKG has been a topic of extraordinary interest in these patients in that they invariably display a completely unique "pseudo-infarction" pattern of posterolateral changes representing a genetically determined focal myocardial scar. In addition, they display so-called "high-frequency notches" (HFN) and tend to have a small number of HFN in the early stages of the disease; with increasing severity of the disease they develop a larger number, and in the terminal stage they again exhibit relatively few notches. It is felt that significant increases or decreases in the count of HFN on QRS complexes can be useful indicators for estimating the extent and severity of cardiac involvement in progressive muscular dystrophy.

---

151. Answer: C

The correct answer is biventricular congestive heart failure. The key to the correct answer here is the noting of left ventricular gallop rhythm and pulmonary edema, thereby implicating LEFT heart failure, as well as right. Acute pulmonary thromboembolism represents, effectively, ACUTE cor pulmonale; cor pulmonale heart disease corresponding more to the COPD patient usually described as the "blue bloater" patient with chronic bronchitis, among others. The choice of pericardial effusion with pericardial tamponade would be unacceptable for the same reason (e.g., failing to account for the left heart failure), but also because there is no data per se presented to support a diagnosis of pericardial disease.

From a test-taker point of view, this is an important point. At this level, tests of this quality are written in such a fashion that one is not expected to invent data that simply is not there, a principle which has its own correlate in the actual practice of medicine, of course.

Eisenmenger's transformation requires a shunt lesion, which is not there; this patient is most often a young adult with a large ventricular septal defect whose torrential left-to-right shunting is converted at least to a balanced shunting phenomenon if not an actual reversal to right-to-left.

152. Answer: E

The correct answer is subxiphoid pericardiostomy with pericardial biopsy. The presence of pulsus paradoxus virtually establishes the diagnosis of hemodynamically significant pericardial tamponade. The treatment principles in this setting include the following:

1) Positive inotropic support
2) (Rapid) Volume infusion
3) Pericardiocentesis under controlled circumstances
4) Pericardiostomy

153. Answer: A

The correct answer is myxomatous mitral valve prolapse. This is the classic "marfanoid" patient with mitral valve prolapse. Patients with the actual autosomal dominant Marfan syndrome of course may have MVP as well, but the typical MVP patient is described herein and will not be a true Marfan patient most of the time. The implications of finding so many relatively tall, lax-jointed young women who may or may not have pectus abnormalities are sizable and suggest some forme fruste of the Marfan spectrum of disease, hence the colloquial term "marfanoid." Personal experience teaches that these patients have an arm span that exceeds their height by 0 to 2 inches, where as the similar comparison in true Marfan patients reveals an arm span exceeding their height by 2 to 4 inches. The metacarpophalangeal pattern profile (MCPP), a radiological method in which the 19 tubular hand bones are assessed, has been used in the diagnosis of various syndromes. Patients with MEN III are often described as "marfanoid" persons with distinctive facial features (bulky lips, thick eyelids) as well as occasional MVP.

Whereas much has been said regarding decisions about endocarditis prophylaxis and MVP, this has helped to inspire the American Heart Association (AHA) to construct a brilliant algorithm in their latest document. There would be no question whatsoever regarding the advisability of traditional precautions in the patient described herein.

154. Answer: C

The correct answer is cor pulmonale due to pulmonary thromboembolism. It is very important to appreciate the fact that ACUTE cor pulmonale represents pulmonary thromboembolism almost by definition. This gentleman may represent another variation on the so-called "economy class syndrome" theme which has been a concern in the commercial air transportation community, although the nature of the association, if any, remains uncertain. Of far more importance in this particular patient may be the neoplasm, the association between a true hypercoagulable state and cancer being well known. This patient has all the features of (acute) pulmonary hypertension and right heart failure. The systemic venous hypertension, as reflected in his jugular venous pulsations, reminds of the important differential diagnosis of this important physical finding, which is:

1) Right heart failure
2) Tricuspid valve disease
3) Pericardial compressive physiology
4) Superior vena cava syndrome

Note that the superior vena cava syndrome patient would have distended, pulseless neck veins as well as the other features that so often accompany the Pancoast tumor, e.g., Horner's syndrome, collar of Stokes, facial suffusion, and a characteristic chest X-ray.

155. Answer: A

The correct answer is normal repolarization variant. Early repolarization (ER), also known as benign early repolarization (BER) or normal variant, is noted in approximately 1% of the population and in up to 48% of patients seen in the ED with chest pain. The electrocardiographic characteristics of ER include widespread ST segment elevation, upward concavity of the initial portion of the ST-segment, notching of the terminal QRS complex, and concordant T waves of large amplitude. The incidence of 1 to 2% is found equally common in all races. The findings are known to regress during exercise testing. The nearly universal impression of an increased frequency in African-American men is not well documented in the literature, although there are very thoughtful statements as to the significance with respect to both thrombolysis criteria and cocaine usage.

156. Answer: B

The correct answer is pulmonary arterial hypertension, acquired via cor pulmonale. In contrast to the patient with pulmonary thromboembolism and ACUTE cor pulmonale, here is the typical picture of CHRONIC cor pulmonale heart disease in the setting of what is no doubt chronic bronchitis. This is the traditional association of the classical 'blue bloater" and the development of pulmonary hypertension, no doubt as a function of the chronic arterial hypoxemia for which they are so well known, although the mechanism is the same in cystic fibrosis.

157. Answer: D

The correct answer is ventricular tachycardia (VT). From a test-taker's point of view, there are seven [7] KEY POINTS in this case, as follows:

1. Older adult
2. Alcohol
3. Syncope
4. Tachycardia at a rate of about 150/min
5. Regular rhythm
6. WIDE QRS complexes
7. Atrioventricular dissociation

With that data base, one is searching for the answer that fits the EKG criteria, which is sufficient to cause syncope, and which the patient could survive long enough to permit the depiction shared by the paramedics. As such, ventricular tachycardia can be the only answer. No one "regains consciousness" during ventricular fibrillation. AV nodal re-entry tachycardia is not wide-complex tachycardia, unless one cares to invoke ventricular aberration, an unnecessary conjecture herein. Multifocal atrial tachycardia is not regular, and sinus tachycardia with bundle branch block would not adequately explain the event.

This question in particular is included in this Practice Set to demonstrate the process of diagnostic clinical reasoning.

The association with alcohol intake is well documented.

158. Answer: D

The correct answer is proximal right coronary artery (RCA). This is the classical picture of inferior myocardial infarction and should correlate with occlusion of a dominant right coronary artery. Worth noting is that 89% of the population have right coronary dominance and hence, a picture like this patient at the time of thrombotic occlusion of that vessel.

159. Answer: A

The correct answer is ostium secundum atrial septal defect (ASD). Again, from a test-taker's point of view, the noting of fixed splitting of the second heart sound means that only one answer is possible on a test. In "real life," there are occasional patients with ventricular septal defect who have this finding, but that would never be the point on an examination of this quality. The flow murmur is typical and represents the shunt volume in the pulmonary artery. In fact, there may be a murmur resulting from the flow across the septal defect itself, but this is in fact a diastolic murmur and is seldom heard clinically.

This phenomenon is also largely exhalation dependent and is therefore, nonetheless, exactly what explains the fixed splitting: Whereas inspiration volume loads the right ventricle in the usual fashion (via acceleration of caval flow), expiration volume loads the right ventricle again (via the increase in shunt volume across the septal defect itself in exhalation), thereby resulting in a balance of loading phenomena affecting the right heart (and effectively "holding" P_2 away from A_2).

160. Answer: C

The correct answer is WPW with orthodromic tachycardia (AVRT). The key to the correct diagnosis here is the noting of the Q-P interval (> 100 msec). In AVNRT, the P-wave is hidden in the QRS complex. These are the patients with congenital dual AV pathways whose re-entry loop is restricted to the area surrounding the AV node. In the patient with AVRT, the normal impulse during tachycardia will travel antegradely down the normal conduction pathway and then will use the Kent pathway for the retrograde limb of the re-entry loop. What this means, however, is that there is a measurably longer distance and greater time needed for the advancing impulse to return to atrial myocardium in order to excite a P-wave, the latter then being delayed and appearing "down the page" in the ensuing ST-segment. Wenckebach (1st degree AV block with Mobitz I progression) would not explain tachycardia, WPW with antidromic tachycardia should be a WIDE-complex tachycardia, and the answer multifocal atrial tachycardia should be irregular. Some authors place the diagnostic threshold of the Q-P interval at shorter levels (e.g., 70 msec).

161. Answer: C

The correct answer is enhanced automaticity. Although not seen on a daily basis, the phenomenon of non-paroxysmal junctional tachycardia is exceedingly important both from a practical clinical point of view as well as a conceptual example. Arguably, this is the very best example of "enhanced automaticity," the junctional tissues having been accelerated non-specifically by one or more of several factors such as the following:

1. Digitalis excess
2. Hypokalemia
3. Post-infarction state
4. Post-operative state
5. Post-prandial hypoglycemia
6. Other

Magnesium sulfate may have a role in treatment, although the usual focus is the correction of the spectrum of reversible contributors operative in the specific patient. The rate-range of 70-130/min is very important, particularly given the overlap with the normal range for the resting sino-atrial node. By way of review, the junctional rhythms are:

##	Name	Rate Range	Significance
1	junctional escape ("idionodal rhythm")	40-60/min	default pacemaker
2	non-paroxysmal junctional tachycardia (NPJT)	70-130/min	as above; never "normal" or "chronic"
3	paroxysmal junctional tachycardia (PJT)	150-250/min	rare, rapid, perhaps "incessant"

162. Answer: D

The correct answer is Adult pattern coarctation of the aorta. The equality of the upper limbs and disparity of the upper versus lower limbs helps identify a narrowing beyond the left subclavian artery, the usual site for the "adult-type" of aortic coarctation. This type is much more common and would be the expected abnormality in this child. The issue of maternal PKU is real and has stimulated the recommendation that if an adult woman has relaxed the diet of her youth, she would want, ideally, to resume the most meticulous diet possible even before conception.

163. Answer: E

The answer is a ventilation/perfusion lung scan showing multiple perfusion defects.

The woman has infective endocarditis of the tricuspid valve, a common occurrence in intravenous drug users. An echocardiogram would be very likely to show a tricuspid vegetation. Given her symptoms and the lung findings, she almost certainly has multiple septic emboli to the lungs, a problem that would be best identified by a ventilation/perfusion lung scan. She has several signs of right heart failure and pulmonary hypertension, but no signs of left heart failure. All of the other choices would reflect left heart failure.

She will need intravenous antibiotics for an extended period of time, and possibly tricuspid valve removal. Some patients do fairly well without a tricuspid valve, but others have refractory peripheral edema, liver congestion, ascites, and so forth. They may require tricuspid valve replacement, usually with a bioprosthetic valve, since mechanical valves have a high thrombosis rate in the tricuspid position. Clearly, any prosthetic valve in an IV drug abuser is subject to reinfection.

164. Answer: E

The answer is no abnormalities.

There has been heightened awareness of sudden death of young people partaking in strenuous exercise after several highly publicized episodes. The largest series of autopsies in these individuals have shown no abnormalities in the majority of patients. Death was presumably due to a ventricular arrhythmia from an unrecognized source, possibly a subclinical cardiomyopathy or an unknown genetic disorder.

If any abnormality is found on autopsy, hypertrophic cardiomyopathy is the most common, followed by anomalous origin of the coronary arteries.

165. Answer: C

The correct answer is a sound heard with the diaphragm at the apex shortly after S2.

This actress was portraying someone with rheumatic mitral stenosis. There would likely be an opening snap heard at the apex after S2. The opening snap is a high-pitched sound, and thus heard better with the diaphragm. S1 is typically loud in mitral stenosis. Aortic regurgitation would produce a decrescendo blowing murmur at the left lower sternal border with the patient sitting forward. Mitral valve prolapse would present with the click and murmur. A sound heard with the bell at the apex after S2 would be an S3, which patients with mitral stenosis are very unlikely to have, since the left ventricle is not filled rapidly.

166. Answer: B

The correct answer is large *a* waves and very large *v* waves.

This person has advanced left and right heart failure from previous myocardial infarctions. Large *a* and *v* waves would be typical of this condition. Large *a* waves and slow *y* descents are associated with tricuspid stenosis. Rapid *x* and *y* descents are found in constrictive pericarditis. Regular cannon *a* waves would occur with the common form of PSVT and ventricular tachycardia with 1:1 retrograde transmission to the atria. In both arrhythmias, atrial and ventricular systole would be simultaneous, producing the cannon *a* waves. Distended non-pulsatile neck veins would be indicative of superior vena caval obstruction, most likely from cancer.

167. Answer: E

The correct answer is acute mitral regurgitation from rupture of a myxomatous chordae. "Joe" has acute severe mitral regurgitation from rupture of a myxomatous chordae of the mitral valve. The clues are the sudden onset of symptoms in an otherwise healthy middle-aged man, the prominent apical impulse (which means this is *not* a left ventricular function problem), and the early systolic decrescendo murmur. Unilateral opacification on a chest x-ray is an uncommon but well-reported presentation of pulmonary edema.

There is no evidence of a myocardial infarction, particularly with the impressive apical impulse and normal electrocardiogram. There cannot be a new VSD because the murmur would be hard to miss, and, again, he has no evidence of an acute infarction. Acute aortic regurgitation could present exactly like this, except that it should produce an early diastolic murmur. Transesophageal echo, had it been available, would have easily have made the correct diagnosis, since the echo image would be unaffected by his mechanical ventilation.

168. Answer: B

The answer is transfer him emergently for mitral valve repair or replacement. This man needs urgent cardiothoracic surgical intervention for the mitral valve. His mortality without immediate surgery is obviously very high. The other choices either are for incorrect diagnoses or delay mitral valve surgery.

169. Answer: D

The answer is a low-pitched mid-diastolic rumble at the apex. These unfortunate women have chronic aortic regurgitation because of syphilitic aortitis. The low-pitched mid-diastolic rumble is the Austin-Flint murmur.

A decreased rise time and volume in the carotid pulses and a late-peaking systolic murmur are features of aortic stenosis. Rapid *y* descents are associated with tamponade. Cyanosis and clubbing indicate either severe pulmonary disease or a congenital cardiac defect.

170. Answer: A

The answer is prescribe sublingual nitroglycerin as needed and begin secondary prevention for coronary artery disease. This man clearly has coronary artery disease. However, it takes an almost heroic amount of exercise to induce symptoms and evidence of ischemia. His exercise results, particularly his long duration of exercise, risk stratify him by the Duke criteria to a 0.25% one-year cardiac mortality. He should receive aggressive secondary prevention, which has a very good chance of making him asymptomatic as well.

He certainly does not need immediate catheterization and revascularization based on his noninvasive test results. Amlodipine is a reasonable choice for treating his hypertension, but it is not part of standard secondary prevention that includes the antihypertensive beta-blockers. There is no need to spend money to obtain further validation of his ischemic heart disease by ordering thallium scintigraphy. Sublingual nitroglycerin is appropriate, but initial therapy with an angiotensin-converting enzyme inhibitor is not part of standard secondary prevention. He has no evidence of left heart failure that would justify the use of this medication.

171. Answer: D

The answer is a ventilation/perfusion lung scan. This complex patient turned out to have normal coronary arteries and pulmonary hypertension. His chronically edematous leg is the source of multiple pulmonary emboli. There is typically a 10-month delay between the onset of symptoms until the diagnosis is made and then only when the patient has advanced pulmonary hypertension. The treatment of this condition was nearly hopeless until pulmonary thromboendarterectomy was developed.

Any type of echocardiogram would show right heart enlargement and pulmonary hypertension, but the latter is obvious from the hemodynamic data. An arterial blood gas might demonstrate hypoxia, but would certainly not be diagnostic. The DL_{CO} would be abnormal, but not specific.

172. Answer: A

The answer is patient A is more likely to have pulsus paradoxus than patient B

These hemodynamic tracings are from patients with tamponade (A) and constrictive pericarditis (B). The only one of the choices that would be expected with tamponade is pulsus paradoxus. The other findings are typical of constriction.

173. Answer: E

The correct answer is treat the immediate pain with an intravenous narcotic and start ibuprofen 2400 mg/day. This woman has atypical chest pain for ischemia and an electrocardiogram that shows diffuse ST segment elevation and PR segment depression, most prominent in lead II. This is the classic ECG for acute pericarditis, and should be treated with pain medications and nonsteroidal anti-inflammatory agents. The worst possible course would be to give thrombolytic therapy, which could result in acute bleeding from the inflamed pericardium and subsequent tamponade.

174. Answer: C

The answer is a 75-year-old man with the onset of chest pain 5 hours ago and a new left bundle branch block. Patients with new left bundle branch block in the clinical setting of an acute ischemic event have the most mortality benefit from thrombolytic therapy because of the amount of myocardium in jeopardy. Patients with anterior ST segment elevation benefit less, with inferior ST segment elevation still less, and are actually harmed with ST segment depression. The 80-year-old woman has a strong indication for thrombolytic therapy except for the recent onset of a neurological deficit. The 72-year-old woman with a tall R wave in leads V_1 and V_2 is having an acute posterior MI and would benefit from thrombolytic therapy to the same extent as an acute inferior MI.

175. Answer: C

The correct answer is inserts a long, large bore needle into her left chest toward her cardiac apex. This poor woman has had severe chest trauma. Her physical neck veins are consistent with acute tamponade, certainly from a traumatic hemopericardium. The chaplain's assistance may be of real use a few hours later. A tension pneumothorax would produce distended pulseless neck veins and absent breath sounds on one side. Rotating tourniquets was an old therapy for heart failure, which she could have conceivably had from coronary artery trauma and myocardial infarction, but the treatment would not have been sufficient.

176. Answer: B

The correct answer is a large, lobulated, mobile mass in the apex of the left ventricle. This poor man had a recent large myocardial infarction and suffered a severe complication. All of the findings point to a severe metabolic acidosis, probably from mesenteric infarction, from an arterial embolism from the apical thrombus. His normal blood pressure alone rules out cardiogenic shock, acute mitral regurgitation, acute ventricular septal defect, and free wall rupture, the four causes of sudden shock post myocardial infarction.

177. Answer: E

The correct answer is aortic dissection can occur in the third trimester of pregnancy without any obvious predisposing factors. Aortic dissections that involve the ascending aorta should always be treated surgically. Appropriate medical therapy is both beta-blockers and nitroprusside. The hemodynamic parameter that is most associated with extension of the dissection is the rate of rise of the aortic pressure. Nitroprusside decreases the aortic systolic pressure, but actually increases the rate of rise because of reflex tachycardia. Beta-blockers and nitroprusside together decrease the rate of rise. Most descending thoracic dissections can be treated medically. Aortic dissection is an uncommon complication of pregnancy, usually occurring in the third trimester. Dissection of the coronary arteries may also occur in pregnant women.

178. Answer: A

The correct answer is aortic regurgitation. Aortic regurgitation tolerates exercise well because exercise does two good things: dilates the peripheral vasculature, allowing more blood to move forward, and tachycardia, which shortens the time for regurgitation during diastole. Exercise is contraindicated in aortic stenosis, hypertrophic cardiomyopathy, and in patients with Eisenmenger's syndrome. Exercise is not dangerous in patients with mitral stenosis, but it is not well tolerated.

179. Answer: A

The correct answer is sudden cessation of the narrow QRS complex tachycardia followed by a 15-second period of asystole. This man has the classic tachycardia-bradycardia syndrome, in which a tachyarrhythmia, in this case the common form of PSVT (producing the regular cannon *a* waves in the neck) stops suddenly as a good reentrant arrhythmia should, and a long pause occurs before the sinus node begins capturing the atrium properly. Careful electrophysiological studies have shown that most of these pauses are caused by SA exit block; that is, the SA node is firing properly but not capturing the atrium. This occurs because of senile infiltration of the conduction system by fibrous tissue, the same cause of most AV nodal and bundle branch blocks. The fibrous tissue is rendered refractory by a supraventricular tachycardia, most frequently atrial fibrillation and atrial flutter, and the patient experiences a long pause that can produce fainting. Treatment involves permanent pacemaker implantation to protect against the bradyarrhythmia, and then whatever treatment is appropriate for the tachyarrhythmia.

There is no reason why this man without evidence of structural heart disease should have ventricular tachycardia. Third degree AV block would be unlikely to occur suddenly upon termination of a supraventricular tachycardia. There is no reason to suspect torsade de pointes. An atrial rate of 330 is very fast for atrial flutter, and this rhythm would not produce regular cannon *a* waves.

180. Answer: C

The correct answer is concentric left ventricular hypertrophy and a left ventricular ejection fraction of 80%. This case represents a common misunderstanding of the hemodynamics of heart failure. This man has severe hypertension but is being treated incorrectly. His chest x-ray indicates that he has a large heart and a high pulmonary capillary wedge pressure, but does not explain the underlying pathophysiology. He has diastolic dysfunction because of the stiffness of his hypertrophied ventricle, but nothing about the physical examination suggests left heart systolic dysfunction or valvular heart disease. He has a prominent apical impulse, indicating an actively contracting left ventricle, and a fourth heart sound caused by his high left ventricular end diastolic pressure. If the proper therapy is not used, he will eventually end up with poor left ventricular function.

181. Answer: A

The answer is stop digoxin, decrease the dose of furosemide, and start beta-blockers. This man needs negative inotropic therapy with beta-blockers or verapamil. He may need some diuretic, but not enough to produce volume depletion and postural hypotension as in this patient. He would need the therapy "Continue digoxin and furosemide, add an angiotensin-converting enzyme inhibitor, low dose carvedilol, and spironolactone" if he had poor left ventricular function. Digoxin has no place in the treatment of a patient with hyperdynamic left ventricular function. The two intravenous inotropic agents are occasionally used for severe end stage systolic heart failure, although they do not have a Class I recommendation for this use.

182. Answer: C

The correct answer is an electrophysiology study. This woman's electrocardiogram shows a short PR interval and a delta wave in several leads, consistent with the Wolff-Parkinson-White syndrome. The modern treatment of patients with symptomatic arrhythmias and WPW is electrophysiology-guided ablation of the accessory pathway. One could argue that an event monitor would be appropriate to show the nature of her arrhythmias prior to going to directly to ablation, but hey, I didn't include that option as one of the choices!

There is no reason why an otherwise healthy young woman needs an echocardiogram or a chest x-ray. She has pseudo-Q waves in the inferior leads and a tall R wave in V_1, suggesting an inferoposterior myocardial infarction, but these are simply the delta waves in those leads. She appears to have left ventricular hypertrophy also, but, again, this finding is not specific with this electrocardiogram. She has not had syncope and has no reason at her age to have atrial fibrillation, so she is unlikely to have the dreaded complication of WPW, deterioration of atrial fibrillation transmitted down the accessory pathway into ventricular fibrillation.

183. Answer: A

The correct answer is contrast chest CT scan. This patient had acute onset of chest pain radiating down his arms. He has a high arched palate on physical exam and a vague family history of his father dying of a "heart attack" at home at age of 45. This patient has Marfan's syndrome and is experiencing an aortic dissection. The best test would be either a transesophageal echo or a contrast chest CT scan. It would be appropriate to follow this patient in the CCU and obtain cardiac enzymes, but before anything else is done he should be evaluated for aortic dissection.

184. Answer: A

The correct answer is trimethoprim/sulfamethoxazole. The combination of Coumadin and TMP/Sulfa can be a very deadly one. It is the most common warfarin (Coumadin) interaction leading to hospitalization in the U.S. Amoxicillin, codeine, and cefixime all do not interact with warfarin (Coumadin). Azithromycin only rarely causes an increase in INR in patients on warfarin. It is not the cause in this case as azithromycin is not a white tablet (it is red).

185. Answer: B

The correct answer is acetaminophen. This patient developed an unexplained increase in her INR. All the choices are drugs that patients can get over the counter or may get from another provider and not report (OCP). The correct answer is acetaminophen, which can increase the INR with as little as 3 extra-strength tablets a day. In one cross-over study, patients on Coumadin who took 4 gm of acetaminophen a day had INRs 1.75 X higher than a group on Coumadin and not taking acetaminophen.

186. Answer: A

The correct answer is gingko biloba. Gingko biloba can increase hemorrhage risk in patients who take it. It can further increase the risk in anticoagulated patients. St. John's wort may increase the metabolism of warfarin and if a patient isn't monitored closely and dose adjusted, use could lead to under-anticoagulation.

187. Answer: D

The correct answer is Guillain-Barré syndrome. Guillain-Barré is the most common inflammatory polyneuropathy. It frequently is preceded by an upper respiratory infection and has been associated with *Campylobacter jejuni* infections as well as EBV, CMV, HIV, mycoplasma, and Lyme disease. Symptoms include an ASCENDING paralysis and AREFLEXIA caused by a segmental demyelination of the peripheral nerves. CSF examination can be helpful and may show an elevated protein with a small increase in CSF WBC. Nerve conduction studies show slowed conduction. Plasmapheresis is useful if it is begun early in the course.

Botulism causes a DESCENDING paralysis and begins with CRANIAL nerve weakness manifested by dysphonia, dysphagia, diplopia, and blurred vision, then followed by the muscle weakness and respiratory insufficiency. Poliomyelitis presents as meningeal symptoms, fever, and asymmetric paralysis. Tick paralysis occurs while the tick is attached and is due to a neurotoxin. It causes an ascending flaccid paralysis and ataxia. Rabies would not be associated with these types of neurologic findings.

188. Answer: A

The correct answer is parvovirus B-19. Parvovirus in AIDS patients has now been classically described as this case illustrates. Patients develop a red cell aplasia with no reticulocyte production. Treatment is with IVIG. The characteristic finding in the bone marrow is GIANT pronormoblasts. Zidovudine could cause anemia but the anemia resolves after stopping the agent. None of the other items mentioned would cause this.

189. Answer: C

The correct answer is blastomycosis. The combination of lung mass, draining cutaneous lesion, and the finding of budding yeast should point you toward either blastomycosis or coccidioidomycosis. Geography will narrow this down to blastomycosis. Histoplasmosis will not usually cause skin lesions as are seen with blastomycosis or coccidioidomycosis. Treatment would be generally with oral itraconazole for about 6 months. If she were severely ill, you would use amphotericin B.

190. Answer: E

The correct answer is itraconazole and its metabolites are below therapeutic levels. The problem with itraconazole (and more so, with ketoconazole) is that an ACID-stomach environment is helpful for absorption. When the patient was placed on ranitidine with his itraconazole, the itraconazole was likely not absorbed. Therefore he has subtherapeutic levels of itraconazole. It is very unlikely that he has *Cryptococcus* now. Itraconazole-resistant *Histoplasma* is likely exceedingly rare. *Candida krusei* is unlikely also. Think about this: If a patient is on FLUCONAZOLE, that is when infections associated with *Candida krusei* will appear on boards and the real world. Yeast that grows in a blood culture or seen on peripheral smear should NEVER be considered a contaminant.

191. Answer: B

The correct answer is parvovirus B-19. Her child had the classic "5th's disease" with slapped cheeks and a serpiginous rash that worsens with heat or sun exposure. She has the classic adult manifestation with joint manifestations. This is yet another manifestation of this virus. Don't forget aplastic anemia, especially in AIDS or sickle cell patients. Human herpes virus 6 causes roseola in kids and is responsible for pneumonia, meningitis, etc. in immunocompromised adults. She doesn't have Lyme disease even though you may have taken the bait with her being from New Lyme, Connecticut (Do you really think I would make it that obvious??). Remember, she's had no fever, no rash. If she had "frank" arthritis also with effusion I'd suspect it more likely. Disseminated gonorrhea in this lady and her child?? That would involve issues that I don't want to get into, plus his rash is not classic for gonorrhea and she has no rash and no evidence of disseminated pustules.

192. Answer: A

The correct answer is *Chlamydia pneumoniae*. The constellation of symptoms--chronic non-productive cough, low-grade fever, hyperemic sore throat, hoarseness--fit this infection. *C. psittaci* is a concern, BUT he has no hepatosplenomegaly. Expect them to give you splenomegaly with this infection. A combination of pneumonia with splenomegaly: think *C. psittaci* or *Coxiella burnetii*!! *Coxiella* I'd also think about if they said he delivered cows or some livestock or more recently CATS have been implicated with this infection—but you have to have contact with placentas usually for this. *S. pneumoniae* is unlikely to produce this prolonged gradual infection and the patchy infiltrate goes against it somewhat. Plus they kept saying he had no chills—if you see "chills" and "rusty sputum" think of *S. pneumoniae*.

193. Answer: D

The correct answer is intravenous penicillin G or ampicillin. This poor woman has bacteremia with *Listeria*, a gram-positive diphtheroid-like organism. Think of this organism if pregnancy is involved or someone who eats a lot of goat or imported cheeses particularly from Mexico. Penicillin or ampicillin is the only thing that will get it reliably. If she is penicillin allergic you could use trimethoprim/sulfamethoxazole. Normally, if you hear about a diphtheroid-like organism you can suspect contamination—however, in someone immunocompromised or semi-immunocompromised (like pregnancy), don't ignore it until you are sure it comes back as something unimportant.

194. Answer: D

The correct answer is to treat again with metronidazole. With *C. difficile* diarrhea it is expected that up to 1/3 of patients may relapse no matter what therapy you use. Therefore repeat therapy with metronidazole is reasonable. Oral vancomycin costs about $300 and is difficult to find. Clindamycin is not an appropriate choice—remember, on a dose-by-dose basis, clindamycin causes *C. difficile* more often than any other antibiotic. BUT, if they ask you which antibiotics cause *C. difficile* diarrhea the most, it is the cephalosporins—because they are used a lot more than other antibiotics. So this is still confusing?? Look at it this way. Which antibiotic (clindamycin or cephalosporin) is more likely to induce *C. difficile* diarrhea in an individual patient? The answer is clindamycin. Which antibiotic nationwide more commonly causes *C. difficile* diarrhea? Cephalosporin. Got it now?

195. Answer: B

The correct answer is azithromycin weekly. Of the choices listed, only the azithromycin weekly is currently approved for prophylaxis. Clarithromycin could be used but he would have to use it daily. Rifampin is not approved for MAI prophylaxis. Rifabutin and clarithromycin would be used for treatment not prophylaxis. The choice of "Nothing" is not correct, as he really is becoming high risk for MAI infection.

196. Answer: C

The correct answer is ceftriaxone and vancomycin. She has pneumococcal meningitis. Realize that in many parts of the United States up to 30% of pneumococci are resistant to penicillin and up to 10% are resistant to the 3rd generation cephalosporins. Know that vancomycin and ceftriaxone are appropriate for presumed pneumococcal meningitis until the sensitivities are known. Another option is ceftriaxone and rifampin. Her prior antibiotic usage increases her risk of having a resistant organism. Ceftazidime is a poor choice as it has diminished gram-positive activity compared to ceftriaxone and cefotaxime. Penicillin alone would be a poor choice because of the high resistant rates. Now, if they tell you the pneumococcus is sensitive to penicillin then that would be the correct choice!

197. Answer: C

The correct answer is *Tropheryma whipplei*. Ok I gave you a hint that this was a hard one. Know this stupid little bug. Patients will present after a LONG time with nonspecific complaints. The main symptoms are weight loss, diarrhea, and arthropathies and in nearly 75% of the cases—these 3 occur together. The GI symptoms usually begin later but frequently lead to the diagnosis. Usually they will present with episodic and watery diarrhea or steatorrhea and are accompanied by abdominal pain and in about 20-30% they will have occult blood in their stool. Skin hyperpigmentation is frequently common to the sun-exposed areas. Just about every organ in the body will be infected with this bacteria. The diagnosis is usually made by upper endoscopy but biopsy of lymph nodes or masses will also yield the diagnosis. Upper endoscopy will show whitish or yellowish plaques distributed on a friable mucosa. The key here is the PAS staining. PCR is also now available and would be useful for confirming this. With PAS staining be careful because a few other conditions in the colon or rectum would show you this—for example, *melanosis coli*. Treatment of this is best with trimethoprim/sulfamethoxazole, but severely ill patients like this guy should receive parenteral ceftriaxone for at least 2 weeks. Amazingly also chloramphenicol (that old antibiotic) would be a good consideration for CNS disease too because of its great penetration. Thus concludes the mini-lecture on this goofy organism that likely will have one question on the ABIM. But, you won't miss it!

198. Answer: B

The correct answer is disseminated *Histoplasma* infection. Note that she has AIDS (or to confirm it we have to wait for the Western blot—but face it; she has an HIV ELISA that is positive, her CD4 count is 37, and she has had sex with a known IV drug abuser). She lives in Memphis, which is endemic for *Histoplasma*. We can rule out Coccidioidomycosis based on her geography. Disseminated *Pneumocystis* is really rare outside of the lung. Lymphoma is possible but less likely given her other findings. Tuberculosis also would be less likely to cause this picture—if she had a higher CD4 count of, say, 300 then we would be more concerned about tuberculosis than an opportunistic infection like *Histoplasma*.

Ok, back to the *Histoplasma*. She has disseminated disease. Likely if we did a bone marrow we would find the organism here. Also, today we can do blood cultures and effectively grow the organism quite easily. The other simple test to do would be to order a serum or urine *Histoplasma* antigen. This is highly sensitive and specific for disseminated *Histoplasma* in HIV-infected patients.

199. Answer: E

The correct answer is herpes simplex meningoencephalitis. The key here is the "bizarre behavior" and the findings on MRI of temporal lobe involvement. To help you diagnose this, a PCR for herpes simplex virus DNA could be helpful on the CSF. CSF cultures for herpes are rarely positive except in the severely immunocompromised or in neonates. He certainly is at risk for syphilis, but the CSF findings don't support it nor does the MRI. You would, though, order a CSF VDRL on this kid just because he is at high risk based on his past history. *Bartonella henselae* is the etiology for Cat Scratch disease and does cause significant CNS disease in children on occasion; usually it will present with seizures, which also is likely with herpes encephalitis too. We have no indication that he has varicella and this does not look like bacterial meningitis with the normal protein and glucose.

200. Answer: C

The correct answer is sucralfate. This agent will substantially interfere with the absorption of the oral drug, resulting in subtherapeutic serum and urine levels. Other agents to avoid that also will do this include antacids that contain magnesium, aluminum, or calcium. Theophylline is another agent to avoid as concurrent ciprofloxacin will cause increases in theophylline levels and possible theophylline toxicity.

201. Answer: A

The correct answer is *Pseudomonas aeruginosa*. This is the most common cause of acute otitis externa in patients with diabetes. Note, this guy needs admission and needs to be treated with intravenous antibiotics that cover *Pseudomonas* well. Choices would include piperacillin/tazobactam or ciprofloxacin. The other choices can cause otitis externa but are less common, especially in diabetics. Oh, the *Streptococcus diabeticus* was something I just made up—sorry, it is Friday afternoon when I'm writing this—I thought I might as well make your day fun too.

202. Answer: D

The correct answer is *Vibrio vulnificus*. This is the classic case to look for on the Boards: An alcoholic man with liver disease who has exposure to salt water or fish and comes in with sepsis and confusion. This is the scenario you should think about for this. Another is if a person with liver disease eats oysters or goes to the beach. The other choices are less likely, particularly Malaria and leptospirosis. Group A *Streptococcus* or a *Staphylococcus* could do this, but his history is too classic to pick anything else but *Vibrio* for this unfortunate man.

203. Answer: C

The correct answer is penicillin G, 3 million units intravenously q 4 hours. This patient has neurosyphilis. But, you say—the CSF VDRL was negative. How can he have neurosyphilis? Because I say so, that's why! Actually, remember that the CSF VDRL is very SPECIFIC (meaning that if it is positive it means they truly have neurosyphilis) but it is not very SENSITIVE (only about half of patients with documented neurosyphilis will have a positive CSF VDRL!!). So you knew he had syphilis, right? The serum VDRL and FTA-ABS were both positive. If you do an LP on someone with neurologic disease and they have a positive RPR or VDRL on their serum that is relatively high, then you are going to have to consider that they might have neurosyphilis. He has meningitis by definition with 50 WBCs in his CSF. And he has an elevated abnormal protein in the CSF. Both go along with neurosyphilis. So, he's got neurosyphilis. And the poor guy also has AIDS too, which he didn't know he had before coming to see you.

Note: Look also for syphilis in a young person with hearing loss!!!!! Always look for syphilis in them!

204. Answer: B

The correct answer is change the catheter site and add amphotericin B. She has infection with *Candida krusei*, which is almost always resistant to fluconazole. Recent literature supports removal and replacement of a central venous catheter if cultures are positive for a *Candida sp.* or other fungemia. NEVER NEVER NEVER consider a *Candida* blood culture result as a contaminant. Remember, with disseminated *Candida* you do want to look for endophthalmitis and liver and splenic lesions, which she did not have at this time. Note that sometimes the liver/spleen lesions may not occur until after her neutropenia has resolved!

205. Answer: D

The correct answer is *Pseudomonas aeruginosa*. Note, he is only 5 days out from his transplant. The most common organisms to cause problems this early are hospital-acquired infections, particularly with gram-negatives like *Pseudomonas*. Note CMV and *Pneumocystis* are likely in 1-4 months out. *Cryptococcus* is a problem more often 4 or more months out. *Legionella* really doesn't have much more increased incidence unless there was something wrong with the processing of water in the hospital.

206. Answer: C

The correct answer is pyrazinamide (PZA). Note that hyperuricemia is common but gout is rare. PZA along with INH and rifampin will cause hepatitis also. INH can cause peripheral neuropathy. Rash is seen with PZA and ethambutol. And with ethambutol the thing to look out for is optic neuritis, particularly manifested by changes in vision, especially with colors.

207. Answer: B

The correct answer is *Bartonella henselae*. This patient has Cat Scratch fever or disease. (Who wrote the song "Cat Scratch Fever"? That's right Ted Nugent.) Note commonly you'll see patients present with axillary nodes and scratches on the hand—that is just too dang easy. But know that a classic conjunctivitis pre-auricular node syndrome is Cat Scratch disease. This is not Lyme disease. This is not herpes. This is really not likely to be MRSA. And the poor turtle here is innocent so *Aeromonas* is not a problem either. Remember for the Boards: Common things are common; rare things are rare. What causes lymph node swelling in a person who works with animals that does not respond to anti-staph drugs?? Most common thing is going to be Cat Scratch.

208. Answer: C

The correct answer is cytomegalovirus retinitis. CMV retinitis is the most common eye disorder to occur in patients with CD4 counts below 50. Patients will frequently initially complain of floaters and gradually they will lose vision. This patient has classic findings on ophthalmologic examination: attenuation of vessels in the area affected by retinitis. Retinal lesions will occur as two possible presentations. In the posterior type, large areas of thick white infiltrate are accompanied by retinal hemorrhage, with a distribution along retinal vessels. The peripheral type demonstrates granular retinitis with satellite lesions and less hemorrhage. Behind the advancing border is necrotic retina. Treatment is with intravenous ganciclovir, foscarnet, or both. Also it is important to get her HIV under better control and with better anti-HIV therapy raise her CD4. This would be very helpful in controlling her disease.

209. Answer: C

MRSE

The correct answer is methicillin-resistant *Staphylococcus epidermidis*. This is a straightforward knowledge question. Remember with prosthetic valve endocarditis that occurs within the first 2 months, methicillin-resistant *Staphylococcus epidermidis* (MRSE) is the most common organism. It also is the most common after 2 months—so that one is easy to remember. Prosthetic valve endocarditis: MRSE. Treatment is with vancomycin + rifampin + gentamicin initially. For native valve endocarditis it gets a little more confusing.

For the non-addict: Divide it into Acute (Usually no previously known valve problem, Janeway lesions) vs. Subacute (usually a previous valvular abnormality, Osler nodes, Roth spots). For Acute, think of *Staphylococcus aureus*. For Subacute, think of the viridans group of *Streptococci* (mouth strep too).

For the addict also divide into acute and non-acute: Acute will be *S. aureus* or *Pseudomonas*. For the subacute, think *Enterococcus*, Viridans type of *Strept* or fungi like *Candida* (particularly for right sided).

For the culture-negative, non-addict think of HACEK, fungal, and weird things like Q fever or *Chlamydia psittaci*.

210. Answer: D

The correct answer is assay for acute and convalescent titers. This patient has (drum roll please) tularemia. To diagnose tularemia, which is due to *Francisella tularensis*, you usually will do acute and convalescent serum titers. You do NOT want to biopsy or aspirate a lymph node with tularemia. You are putting yourself and the lab at risk for aerosolization of the organism. Febrile agglutinins are WORTHLESS. CAN I SAY IT STRONGER? NEVER EVER ORDER febrile agglutinins on anybody on the ABIM!! Treatment of this man would be with either IM streptomycin, IV gentamicin, or oral doxycycline. He doesn't appear to be that ill so oral doxycycline might be worth a trial. There is a higher risk of relapse with oral doxycycline though.

211. Answer: B

The correct answer is ehrlichiosis. This patient has fever and non-specific symptoms. He has splenomegaly. He has pancytopenia with elevated liver transaminases. This picture goes with ehrlichiosis. For tularemia, you would expect lymphadenopathy and not expect to find a pancytopenia. *Histoplasma* and blasto would be unusual to present in this fashion. This also is not a presentation for Lyme disease.

212. Answer: A

The correct answer is *Neisseria gonorrhoeae*. Ms. Smith has the classic findings of disseminated gonorrhea. Note, if she was having her menses that would have been even more indicative of this type of infection. Remember that women are more likely to have this than men. It is unlikely that you will grow the organism from the blood but possibly from the genitourinary tract. The other thing to remember is that ceftriaxone is the treatment of choice because of the resistance problem with penicillin in the United States. None of the other choices would fit this picture except for possibly *Streptococcus pyogenes* but endocarditis would have to be in the differential and she has no evidence of this from the history—she is just a very "active" woman with no history of IV drug abuse.

213. Answer: D

The correct answer is *Mycobacterium tuberculosis*. He most likely has AIDS. He has scattered lymphadenopathy with lower lobe infiltrates. He does not have severe hypoxia or disseminated diffuse disease on CXR helping to differentiate from *Pneumocystis*. The hilar adenopathy helps you lean toward tuberculosis also. The other organisms are much less likely. Look for *Bartonella* with skin lesions; *Rhodococcus* is possible but much rarer than *Mycobacterium tuberculosis*. He has no travel history to suggest that coccidioidomycosis should be considered.

214. Answer: A

The correct answer is oral fluconazole. She has a cystitis with a yeast likely to be sensitive to fluconazole and more than likely due to the stupid urethral catheter that should have been removed days ago. You would not subject this woman to amphotericin (ampho-terrible) B and oral administration only works for oral and esophageal candidiasis. Re-insertion of the in-dwelling urethral catheter is not a good idea because you will likely just perpetuate her symptoms with continued colonization of her bladder.

215. Answer: B

The correct answer is to call for an immediate ENT or Anesthesia consultation and start ceftriaxone now. This patient has acute epiglottitis. The usual organisms are *Haemophilus influenzae* and more recently *Streptococcus pyogenes*. Classically this was a disease of childhood but with *H. influenzae* immunization, this disease has decreased markedly in incidence. The other antibiotic choices are not good choices for *H. influenzae*. The choice of initially culturing the throat is definitely a no-no. You should do as little as possible in manipulation of the oropharynx. Frequently you don't even want to look in the mouth if it will upset the patient. That is why immediate ENT or anesthesia back up is needed for protection of the patient's airway.

216. Answer: C

The correct answer is HIV ELISA. Patients with HIV infection have an increased risk of having recurrent infections with *Salmonella* particularly *S. typhimurium*. KNOW THIS: If someone has recurrent bacteremias with *Salmonella typhimurium* or *Streptococcus pneumoniae* think about HIV! Another little tidbit: If they give you someone from Southeast Asia and they are growing *Penicillium marneffei,* then also think about HIV. The other choices are much less likely to be helpful in this patient. Be aware also that complement deficiency can predispose to these infections too; as well as sickle cell patients and others without functional spleens.

217. Answer: D

The correct answer is *Clostridium tetani*. This man has TETANUS!! Look for it in elderly people who have likely not been immunized in years. Classically they will present with "lockjaw" and then progress to have the other symptoms. The weird opisthotonic posturing described is classic for tetanus. Note, that the only other thing that will do this is strychnine poisoning. Dystonic reactions to drugs can also look like this, but remember that usually this involves LATERAL HEAD TURNING, which is very rare in tetanus. Dental infections may produce trismus but do not cause the other manifestations of tetanus. Treatment is well laid out in many texts: Always protect the airway, administer diphenhydramine to be sure you are not dealing with a dystonic reaction; then proceed to giving a benzodiazepine to control spasms and decrease rigidity. Treatment consists of administering human tetanus immunoglobulin and immunization with Td (tetanus toxoid). Metronidazole is also given for 7-10 days. The course can be quite prolonged and require 6-8 weeks of intense rehabilitative therapy. Patients will receive 3 Td doses over the period of 8 weeks.

218. Answer: A

The correct answer is begin Combivir (zidovudine/lamivudine) and nevirapine. She most likely has HIV-related immune thrombocytopenia—this is very COMMON in HIV-infected individuals. Treatment with combination therapy has shown to be most effective (especially those using zidovudine). Steroids would be contraindicated in this immunocompromised patient and we have no evidence that parvovirus B-19 might be involved with a severe anemia, so use of IVIG is also not warranted. She is not actively bleeding and her platelet count is above 20,000, so there is no need to transfuse her with platelets at this time. If you see pancytopenia, think of an opportunistic disease.

219. Answer: B

The correct answer is *Yersinia enterocolitica*. I don't know if they will ask about this or not—but just in case I threw this question in. There has been a lot of literature about transfusion-related infections—most commonly they are due to Pseudomonas, BUT recently there have been well-documented cases due to *Yersinia enterocolitica*. This organism grows in high concentrations in stored, packed red cells because of contamination by an asymptomatic donor with bacteremia. The organism grows well at the temperature blood is stored and grows really well in the presence of iron and dextran! This may be too esoteric for the general IM boards, but I just have a feeling they might have something about this as one of their "toughie" questions. Now you won't miss it.

220. Answer: E

The correct answer is to continue INH, repeat serum aminotransferase measurements in one month or sooner if clinically warranted. Remember that these values can go up to 3 x normal WITH SYMPTOMS and 5 x normal WITHOUT SYMPTOMS!! before you worry about stopping or changing agents. Also, the current guidelines published in June of 2000 in the MMWR vol .49; no RR-6 state that routine testing is NOT recommended unless patients have a history of liver disease, have HIV infection, are pregnant, are immediately postpartum (within 3 months of delivery), drink alcohol regularly, take other medications that have potential liver toxicity effects, or are at risk for chronic liver disease.

221. Answer: C

The correct answer is hepatitis B vaccine and hepatitis B immune globulin. The mother is most likely a carrier with hepatitis B infection. She can pass this to her newborn infant at delivery and therefore the child should receive both hepatitis B immune globulin as well as vaccine within the first 12 hours of birth! They should be given in two separate sites also. This is true for any instance in which you are giving an "immune globulin" type product and the vaccine concurrently. Otherwise the immune globulin will "bind up" the vaccine and prevent an immunologic response from occurring in the recipient of the vaccine. Note that this scenario would also work for someone who was exposed to a person with hepatitis B—as with a sexual exposure or a needlestick exposure.

Note also that if the exposed person has received vaccine and is known to be immune, you don't have to do anything as that is the purpose the vaccine—it will protect the exposed person.

222. Answer: C

The correct answer is *Mycobacterium marinum*. Think about this organism in someone who is around water and marine organisms. For humans, the most common method of getting this is minor trauma, particularly contact with fish spines or crustaceans. The infection takes awhile to incubate, usually 2-3 weeks and obviously will not respond to routine antibiotics. Sporotrichosis, chromomycosis, and blastomycosis can also all present like this—but nothing in the history helps us think about these. *Vibrio vulnificus* is also associated with water BUT you would expect to see BULLOUS skin lesions and it is usually seen in someone with liver disease, particularly alcoholics.

Oh yeah, Bartonella Crustacea does not exist (yet) and there is no such thing as Crab Scratch fever—until a new Ted Nugent decides to write that one.

223. Answer: E

The correct answer is herpes simplex virus. Even though this man has been in an area with possible tularemia, it is very unlikely to present in this fashion. He has not been in an endemic area for Lyme disease (*Borrelia burgdorferi*). *Listeria* and *Streptococcus* are much less likely based on his CSF findings. The protein and glucose are normal, which indicates more likely a viral etiology. Also, his confusion indicates encephalitis is also occurring, which more commonly occurs with herpes infection than with any of the other organisms listed.

224. Answer: C

The correct answer is fluoroscopic guided aspiration of the hip. You need to attempt to get an organism before starting therapy. It is likely to be *Staphylococcus* but could be either methicillin-sensitive or resistant and other organisms are possible because a previous surgery is involved. This is a chronic problem and blood cultures are likely not to be helpful. The bone scan really is not of any help either—we know he has bone involvement by plain films. Starting therapy at this point is not prudent and it is probable that he will need removal of the prosthesis and debridement of the area.

225. Answer: A

The correct answer is enterotoxigenic *Escherichia coli*. She has "Montezuma's revenge." This is usually a non-bloody diarrhea that resolves without treatment. Eating leafy vegetables or uncooked foods will expose travelers to this organism. Additionally, ice and water are another common source, as travelers mistakenly think that ice is protected. Also, a few people feel like the alcohol in a mixed drink will kill the bacteria—sorry, it doesn't work that way. The other bacteria listed would generally cause much longer symptoms and more extensive disease. Remember with *E. coli* 0157:H7 NOT to give antibiotics—this is new from several reports in the NEJM in recent years. Rotavirus is unlikely and you would expect it more often in a day-care setting or with exposure to children.

226. Answer: C

The correct answer is neurocysticercosis. This term is used for human CNS infection with *Taenia solium* cysts. Most literature involves intracerebral cysts that produce seizures and mass effects. Intraventricular cysts as well as subarachnoid cysts can also occur. Drug therapy with albendazole is the treatment of choice. Sometimes corticosteroids are also required if CNS inflammation is severe or causing symptoms. He does not have HIV, so that really throws *Toxoplasma* and *Cryptococcus* out the window. Lymphoma would be really unusual to give you "cystic" lesions. HSV should not do this normally.

Also, with this think of someone with seizures who has this lesion but they haven't traveled anywhere. The kicker is that they live with a housekeeper or someone who has the infection and is transmitting it fecally/orally in the house. Usually it is a cook or something like that. Lots of literature on this in the early 1990s, so be aware of the "cook" from Mexico and the kid or the mother who starts to have a seizure disorder after a year or two.

227. Answer: D

The correct answer is *Staphylococcus aureus*. Note that this is a toughie unless you put everything together. "Mucous membrane changes; hypotension; rash; renal involvement, liver involvement, hematologic involvement." What gives you hypotension with a rash and multi-organ involvement with a history of trauma?? Toxic Shock Syndrome!! And that is what this poor man has. Change the dog bite to say a scratch from a piece of metal or a post-op patient after surgery. Now does it make more sense?? The dog bite may have tricked you, but remember he is NOT immunocompromised. This guy is a normal dude. Disseminated *Pasteurella* and *Eikenella* are really unusual and unlikely to give you this constellation of findings—endocarditis, yes—but multi-organ involvement, no. *Bartonella henselae* (Cat Scratch) would not do this either. That leaves *Neisseria* and it is possible, BUT the trauma history is what should have led you to *Staphylococcus*. I told you this one is hard…BUT when you get someone with multi-organ involvement and a RASH, think of toxic shock syndrome—either due to *Staphylococcus* or *Streptococcus pyogenes*!!

Remember the difference between these two: with *Staphylococci* you rarely culture the organism in the blood; with *Streptococcus* you are more likely to.

228. Answer: E

The correct answer is False-positive HIV ELISA for HIV-1. She never should have been told she had HIV infection. False-positive HIV ELISAs are quite common; that is why we must wait for the Western blot results. Unfortunately, indeterminate Western blots are also seen occasionally. They generally are false-positive results and are positive in only 1 band that is tested. The other thing to note is that this patient is really at low risk. When you test a low-risk population with a highly sensitive test you are likely to see a large number of false-positive test results. It was possible early on that this was early HIV-1 infection; however, by 3 months and 6 months she should have developed more bands. Resolved HIV infection in adults has not been clinically described. HIV-2 infection would show up on the Western blot. The other choice that this is a false-negative Western blot is very unlikely at this point.

229. Answer: A

The correct answer is mefloquine, starting one week before his travel and continuing for 4 weeks after returning to the U.S. This is a standard question. Mefloquine is the drug of choice. Remember to start it a week before leaving and continuing for 4 weeks after returning from an endemic area. Chloroquine resistance is too high in

Africa to consider its use. Doxycycline for that prolonged period of time in a person who will be exposed to sunlight a lot is not practical from a gastrointestinal standpoint or sunburn standpoint. Primaquine is not used for prophylaxis but is used as an adjuvant treatment for *Plasmodium ovale* and *vivax* to get rid of the "liver" forms of this disease.

230. Answer: C

The correct answer is Papanicolaou smear, RPR, HIV counseling, GC, and *Chlamydia* culturing. Note that HSV culturing is not likely to be helpful. If she is asymptomatic you would not treat her even if she had positive cultures and it would not be causing her discharge. Culturing for *Gardnerella* is not cost-effective, is difficult to do, and likely would not yield meaningful results. *Candida* culturing is not going to be helpful. She likely is colonized, and so even if you find the organism it doesn't necessarily mean that it is causing the problem. You must determine if she has gonorrhea or *Chlamydia*. Both are treatable diseases and it is important for her to know and for the public health officials in the community to be aware of either of these infections so that partner notification can occur.

231. Answer: E

The correct answer is No prophylaxis is indicated. Note that urine is not on the list of body fluids to be worried about with transmission. Blood, semen, vaginal secretions, CSF, synovial, pleural, peritoneal, pericardial, and amniotic fluid are considered "potentially infectious fluids." Let's say this was blood in a cup. Mr. Bore would have exposure to blood of large volume to what would be considered "skin with integrity potentially compromised." The source patient's HIV viral load is really high so we would offer Mr. Bore the three-drug therapy listed of zidovudine, lamivudine, and indinavir for 4 weeks. No data exists (at least as of October 2002) on whether you should change therapy based on genotypes. Some authorities currently recommend considering it, but for Board purposes they won't ask you this. Remember, for large amounts of infectious fluid exposure with a high viral load to use 3-drug prophylaxis! For non-infectious fluid or fluid that is only in contact with "intact skin only" no prophylaxis is indicated.

232. Answer: B

The correct answer is *Bacillus cereus*. Let's "be serious" for a moment (Ok, bad ID joke.) This is an obvious emergency and this organism is a bad one. It is associated with penetrating injury to the eyeball. Remember also that is causes food–poisoning, particularly the "Chinese rice bowl" variety. *Acanthamoeba* is associated with contact lenses and solutions, so think about that if they give you a patient with that type of scenario. *Staphylococcus epidermidis*—think about after ocular surgery—particularly cataract extraction or lens implantation. It can also occur after trauma, but *B. cereus* is one of the few that will give you a ring abscess: Pseudomonas and Proteus are about the only other two agents that will do that as well. *Bartonella henselae*—no kitties around in the history and usually you'll get a conjunctivitis picture, NOT this nasty scenario. So just remember penetrating eye injury with ring abscess formation in the cornea: *B. cereus*!

233. Answer: B

The correct answer is cefotetan. Ingestion of alcohol by patients receiving cephalosporins containing the MTT (methylthiotetrazole) moiety at position 3 has been associated with disulfiram-like reactions. The MTT group's configuration is similar to disulfiram, and appears to block alcohol metabolism at the acetaldehyde step. The accumulation of acetaldehyde is associated with these symptoms. The antibiotics with the MTT side group are cefotetan, cefamandole, cefoperazone, moxalactam, and cefmetazole. Note that these agents also inhibit vitamin K 2,3—epoxide reductase, which converts inactive vitamin K to its active form. Therefore, in a patient with already depleted vitamin K (like an alcoholic or someone with liver disease) use of these antibiotics could increase the PT and cause bleeding problems.

234. Answer: E

The correct answer is further evaluation for depression and referral for counseling. Mr. Benois has classic signs of depression with change in sleeping and eating patterns and loss of interest in usual entertaining activities. EBV serology has been blamed for many things, from chronic fatigue to a persistent EBV syndrome. So far most medical literature does not support this agent as a culprit for these syndromes. He has a completely normal examination. You have no documentable symptoms except his fatigue and he has had major life complications in the past year. These patients can be very difficult to convince that depression could be at the root of their problem. Frequently it takes a combination of medication as well as an effective counselor to help these patients get back to a normal life. After starting Mr. Benois on an antidepressant and receiving counseling he returned to his youthful healthy self; lost 30 lbs in 6 months and was remarried 3 years later. Not all patients are success stories like this, but it should be remembered that a non-specific laboratory test, if misinterpreted, can frequently cause more harm than good.

235. Answer: A

The correct answer is trimethoprim/sulfamethoxazole. This patient with advanced HIV disease develops hyperkalemia while being treated for PCP. TMP/Sulfa can block tubular potassium secretion and severe hyperkalemia has been reported in AIDS patients receiving IV TMP/Sulfa for the treatment of PCP. Hyperkalemia has also been reported in elderly patients receiving oral TMP/Sulfa. Although adrenal insufficiency can cause hyperkalemia and does occur in patients with advanced HIV disease, it would be unlikely in this patient because he received steroids (Solu-Medrol).

236. Answer: B

The correct answer is no therapy at this time. This patient is asymptomatic but has a positive urine culture for a frequently drug-resistant organism. Most chronically catheterized patients will have positive urine cultures. Treatment should only occur if the patient has a symptomatic infection. This patient is asymptomatic, including a normal WBC. Attempted treatment would likely lead to a more drug-resistant organism without offering benefit to the patient.

237. Answer: C

The correct "incorrect" answer is responsible for increased renin in hypertensive subjects. Converting enzyme inhibitors are effective antihypertensive agents, with rare side effects of cough (10%), reversible renal insufficiency, hyperkalemia, and angioedema (<0.1%). They have been proven effective in slowing the rate of progression of diabetic and other proteinuric renal diseases. Discontinuation rates for hyperkalemia are low (<1% in studies). Patients with renal artery stenosis often have an exaggerated response to converting enzyme inhibitors. Renin levels are high in patients taking these agents.

238. Answer: B

The correct answer is her total body sodium is approximately normal. In a hyponatremic patient, low urine osmolality always diagnoses psychogenic polydipsia. Treatment is supportive and while hypertonic saline should be considered in symptomatic patients with hyponatremia, this hyponatremia will likely resolve at a rapid rate with fluid restriction alone. In fact, if chronic, water therapy is sometimes needed to keep the rate of correction at <2mEq/l/hour. Diuretic abuse will lead to a higher urine osmolality when not in use or a higher urine sodium when in use. High ADH levels lead to a concentrated urine. While the patient's volume status is mildly expanded from water, total body sodium is regulated normally and kept negligibly lower than normal.

239. Answer: E

The correct answer is alkalinization of the urine. Rhabdomyolysis classically presents as acute renal failure with pigment in the urine in excess of red blood cells, muddy brown casts, and disproportionate increases in creatinine compared to BUN. Alcohol and cocaine use are often precipitating factors. Treatment includes optimization of volume status and a forced alkaline diuresis, if possible. No indications for dialysis have arisen, the hypocalcemia (or hyperkalemia) does not warrant emergent therapy as intracellular stores may be released later and the high phosphorus is also a cause for hypocalcemia that should not be treated aggressively with calcium (may precipitate metastatic calcification). The patient is hyponatremic and does not need free water replacement at this time.

240. Answer: B

The correct answer is low calcium diet. Stone formation in a patient with hypokalemia, an anion gap acidosis with a high urine pH, positive urine anion gap, and family history of stones suggests Type I RTA (distal). Abnormal growth may also be seen. Bicarbonate or citrate therapy corrects the acidosis and citrate corrects the associated hypocitraturia; fluid therapy helps prevent stones. Thiazide therapy might help limit stone formation but might exacerbate hypokalemia. Low calcium diets are of no value in this setting.

241. Answer: A

The correct answer is renal artery stenosis. Alkalosis is generated when acid is lost or excess bicarbonate is generated in the kidney. It is then maintained by ongoing proximal reclamation and distal acidification driven by aldosterone. Chloride depletion contributes in vomiting, contraction, prior diuretic use, and is diagnosed by a low urine chloride (<10 mEq/L). Severe hypokalemia can lead to a chloride-resistant alkalosis, but this is more commonly seen with hyperaldo states such as renal artery stenosis, licorice intake, or primary hyperaldosteronism.

242. Answer: D

The correct answer is high dose steroids and cytotoxic drugs. This patient has a representative presentation of vasculitis with weight loss, fevers, acute glomerulonephritis, and a + P-ANCA, likely representing microscopic PAN. The renal biopsy is consistent with a pauci immune necrotizing GN, typical of mPAN. Treatment consists of high dose steroids and cytotoxic drugs, usually cyclophosphamide. Imuran has not proven effective and steroids alone are inadequate; bedrest and diuretics might help the blood pressure but also are inadequate therapy. The role of ACEI has not been studied and plasmapheresis appears ineffective.

243. Answer: C

The correct answer is cause hypercalcemia in some users. Loop diuretics inhibit the Na, K 2 Cl transporter leading to natriuresis, kaliuresis, and reduction in blood pressure. They enhance proximal sodium reabsorption leading to alkalosis and increases in uric acid, occasionally precipitating gout. They are associated with calcium and magnesium losses, and are used in the treatment of significant hypercalcemia.

244. Answer: B

The correct answer is that cyclosporine can cause acute and chronic renal damage by means of vasoconstriction. Cyclosporine works by inhibiting T cell function and inhibiting production of interleukin 2. It does not cause pancytopenia. There are multiple drug interactions to be concerned about, and toxicities include renal dysfunction due to vasoconstriction, hypertension, hyperkalemia, gout hirsutism, neurotoxicity, and infection. However, the incidence of infection in cyclosporine-treated patients is no greater than that of patients taking azathioprine and steroids for their immunosuppression.

245. Answer: E

The correct answer is enalapril. Multiple studies have demonstrated reduction in proteinuria with ACE inhibitors and increasing studies are demonstrating enhanced renal survival as well as enhanced cardiac survival with these agents. A biopsy is generally unrewarding as the specificity of a diagnosis of diabetic nephropathy approaches 100% when patients have proteinuric renal insufficiency and retinopathy. Renal artery stenosis is unlikely in this case. Dihydropyridines appear inferior to ACEI in studies and may exacerbate proteinuria. Weight loss, sugar control, and low-salt diets are reasonable, but are not the mainstay of therapy.

246. Answer: A

The correct answer is cryoglobulinemia. Patients with HCV are at significant risk of developing GN. They develop circulating immune complexes and can have cryoglobulinemia. They also have MPGN with low complements in the absence of cryos. More rarely these patients can have membranous nephropathy. In this case, the nephritic presentation, hypocomplementemia, and lack of cryoglobulins suggest MPGN; membranous and FSGS are nephrotic disorders, and they and IgA nephropathy are normal complementemic.

247. Answer: D

The correct answer is acute renal failure secondary to rhabdomyolysis associated with hypophosphatemia. This patient has alcoholic ketoacidosis (AKA) and presents with the classic constellation of findings of alcohol binging, hypoglycemia, and an anion gap metabolic acidosis. These patients usually have hypophosphatemia, which can be severe, and hypomagnesemia. The hypophosphatemia can be severe enough to result in rhabdomyolysis. The diagnosis of alcoholic ketoacidosis may be missed as these patients improve quickly with glucose administration and the ketones are initially beta- hydroxybutyrate and are not detected in the serum until they are converted to acetoacetate. Recognition of the clinical syndrome allows one to monitor and appropriately replace phosphorus early in the hospitalization to prevent complications such as rhabdomyolysis.

Note that acute renal failure secondary to ethylene glycol intoxication is incorrect. The most important clue to the diagnosis of either ethylene glycol or methanol intoxication is an osmolar gap greater than 10. The osmolality is calculated as 2 x sodium + glucose/18+ BUN/2.8. This value will be significantly greater than the measured osmolality in patients with alcohol, methanol, or ethylene glycol ingestion. Also in patients with ethylene glycol ingestion, calcium oxalate crystals may be present in the urine, a rather important clue on board exams. Treatment includes ethanol administration, thiamine, and pyridoxine.

For the answer of methanol intoxication, an osmolar gap is usually present along with an anion gap acidosis. These patients typically present with a fruity odor and blurred vision due to the degradation of methanol to formaldehyde and formic acid, which is toxic to the optic nerve. Treatment includes ethanol administration and hemodialysis.

Isopropyl alcohol is metabolized to acetone and may result in ketosis; however, this patient does not have an acidosis.

The diagnosis of hepatorenal syndrome should be suspected in patients with cirrhosis, portal hypertension, and ascites. Patients who develop acute renal failure in this setting must be evaluated for intravascular volume depletion, frequently associated with diuretics, vomiting, or bleeding or they may develop acute renal failure associated with acute tubular necrosis associated with many of the medications they receive. The diagnosis of HRS depends on demonstrating a benign urinalysis, extremely low fractional excretion of sodium, no response to volume repletion, and exclusion of obstruction or toxic causes.

248. Answer: D

The correct answer is to begin therapy with recombinant human erythropoietin. In patients with diabetic nephropathy, the cornerstone of therapy is control of hypertension with an ACE inhibitor or an ARB. At the present time, there is not enough data to definitely recommend combinations of these drugs. However, management of anemia in these patients is important, as anemia contributes both to progression of renal disease and to cardiovascular disease. The target hemoglobin in patients with chronic renal failure and those with end-stage renal disease is 11-12. Patients with values below this level should be initiated on erythropoietin therapy once it has been confirmed that adequate iron studies are present. Recommendations for adequate iron are an iron saturation greater than 20% and a ferritin greater than 100. In this patient, it would be appropriate to initiate therapy with subcutaneous outpatient erythropoietin.

To refer the patient for renal biopsy to exclude other causes of nephrotic syndrome is incorrect. The diagnosis of diabetic nephropathy is almost always established on clinical grounds alone. Long-standing diabetes associated with retinopathy, nephropathy, hypertension, and even neuropathy in the absence of another obvious cause is adequate to make a clinical diagnosis and therefore no biopsy is necessary. The most important aspect of evaluation in considering other causes in this patient would be the history and physical examination, and without evidence of other systemic disease in a patient with long-standing diabetes, workup is necessarily limited. However, patients who develop renal disease with only a short history of diabetes, absence of retinopathy, signs or symptoms of a systemic disease, or a "nephritic" presentation require more extensive evaluation.

There are no indications for dialysis present in this patient. While early referral of diabetics is important, particularly if they are to receive a vascular access, there are no indications to initiate dialysis in this patient. The classic manifestation of uremia begins with malaise, loss of appetite, weight loss, and progress to nausea, vomiting, and eventual encephalopathy. Patients with significant renal failure who develop symptomatic volume overload, or hyperkalemia, should be considered for urgent dialysis, both of which generally do not occur until the GFR is less than 10 ml/minute, in most patients. The calculated GFR, using the creatinine clearance in this patient, is around 20 ml/minute.

To discontinue lisinopril is incorrect – both ACE inhibitors and angiotensin 2 receptor blockers are cornerstones in the treatment of diabetic nephropathy. Concern is frequently raised when these drugs are administered in patients whose creatinine is rising. In patients with angiotensin II-dependent renal function, i.e., those with perfusion abnormalities due to either severe congestive heart failure or bilateral renal artery stenosis, these agents may reduce glomerular capillary pressure and therefore reduce GFR by blocking A-II. However, in patients with chronic renal failure that is slowly progressive, typical of diabetes, the benefits of these agents strongly outweigh the risks and therefore these agents should be administered in the setting of not only diabetes but other causes of chronic renal failure. The important limiting factor is frequently the potassium, which can be a greater problem in diabetics who are more likely to have underlying Type IV renal tubular acidosis.

To administer a nonsteroidal anti-inflammatory drug to reduce proteinuria is not correct. While there are some studies that have shown that NSAIDs may reduce proteinuria in the setting of nephrotic syndrome, they are likely to cause a predictable decrease in the GFR in these patients and they may also interfere with potassium excretion. Patients with nephrotic syndrome depend on vasodilating prostaglandins to maintain adequate renal perfusion. NSAIDs administered to patients with edema-forming states, such as nephrotic syndrome or cirrhosis, may result in an acute decrease in the GFR and also increase sodium reabsorption, which exacerbates the underlying condition. Because nonsteroidals interfere with sodium excretion in the proximal tubule, there is less sodium delivered to the distal tubule for exchange with potassium, therefore increasing the likelihood of hyperkalemia as well. NSAIDs should therefore not be administered in patients with nephrotic syndrome.

249. Answer: B

The correct answer is a CT scan of the renal veins. Nephrotic syndrome is associated with a hypercoagulable state due to the loss of antithrombin 3, and patients with membranous glomerulopathy are at higher risk for the development of renal vein thrombosis. This diagnosis should be considered in patients who have severe nephritic syndrome and in whom hematuria, flank pain, or acute deterioration of renal function develops. However, more often patients are asymptomatic, and a high index of suspicion is necessary in predisposed patients. Diagnosis can be made noninvasively using CT or MRI, though angiography has been the traditional way to confirm a diagnosis. If acute, patients should receive thrombolytic therapy, though all patients will require chronic anticoagulation.

It is incorrect to initiate therapy with prednisone. This patient has had a sudden deterioration of renal function, which is not the typical course for membranous glomerulopathy. Acute therapy of the underlying disease is therefore less likely to be effective and prednisone alone is not the most effective protocol that is currently being used. Successful protocols using steroids with either chlorambucil or cyclophosphamide have been published, but the most effective therapeutic protocol remains controversial.

To obtain urgent angiography to exclude bleeding from the renal biopsy is incorrect also. While hematuria is a known complication following renal biopsy, this generally occurs within two weeks of the procedure and, when severe, is typically accompanied by flank pain. Painless hematuria four months following a biopsy would be extremely unusual. Initial screening tests would be a noninvasive imaging procedure, such as either an ultrasound or preferably CT scan, which would demonstrate a hematoma of the involved kidney. These patients typically have an acute fall in the hemoglobin as well.

It is unnecessary to refer the patient to a hepatologist for interferon therapy for hepatitis B. Reports have demonstrated that patients with membranous glomerulopathy secondary to hepatitis B may have resolution of the nephrotic syndrome following appropriate treatment of hepatitis B in clearing of the antigen. This would be appropriate in patients with symptomatic disease and evidence of active liver disease. The rapid deterioration of this patient's renal function cannot be explained on the basis of her hepatitis B.

Finally, urology consultation is not required. As in all cases of hematuria, one must determine whether this bleeding is upper or lower urinary tract. Given the patient's history of nephritic syndrome, one would be more concerned about renal vein thrombosis than a new urologic problem which would have to be bilateral or in the bladder to cause such a rise in the creatinine.

250. Answer: C

The correct answer is water retention. – In patients with severe congestive heart failure with marked reduction of cardiac output, both the renin angiotensin aldosterone system and antidiuretic hormone are stimulated. Stimulation of ADH results in water retention. This condition also occurs in patients with severe nephrotic syndrome or cirrhosis. Fractional excretion of sodium will be low and patients require treatment with water restriction, diuretics, and sodium restriction.

An incorrect response is renal sodium losses secondary to furosemide. Hyponatremia is related more to water retention from excess ADH than due to sodium losses. Both furosemide and thiazide diuretics may cause hypovolemia, stimulating ADH and renal retention of water, which results in hyponatremia. Life-threatening hyponatremia has been reported in patients recently started on thiazide diuretics due to a reduction in the diluting capacity of the kidney and increased ADH release, associated with severely restricted Na intake.

SIADH is incorrect. Diagnosis of SIADH cannot be made in the face of heart failure, renal disease, adrenal disease, or volume depletion. Patients with SIADH are normo-volemic and demonstrate a urine osmolality that is inappropriately high when compared with the serum osmolality. One clue to the diagnosis frequently is hypouricemia.

Adrenal insufficiency is incorrect also. Adrenal insufficiency should be considered in all patients who present with hyponatremia and hypovolemia with an elevated urine sodium. The lack of mineralocorticoid production results in sodium wasting by the kidney and may be associated with hyperkalemia and metabolic acidosis.

The choice of hypothyroidism is incorrect. Hypothyroidism causes water retention and patients remain euvolemic. Urine sodium will be elevated. This diagnosis should always be considered when SIADH is also suspected.

251. Answer: B

The correct answer is urine eosinophils. In hospitalized patients who develop acute renal failure, one must always consider medications as the cause. In this patient, the administration of trimethoprim/sulfamethoxazole should raise the possibility of acute interstitial nephritis. Acute interstitial nephritis is a hypersensitivity reaction that frequently produces eosinophilia in the serum and eosinophils in the urine; however, patients may still have AIN even in the absence of this finding. More recently, Hansel stain has been shown to be most effective in demonstrating eosinophils, though Wright stain has traditionally been used. The most common medications that cause acute interstitial nephritis are the non-steroidal anti-inflammatory drugs, and antibiotics including sulfa-based antibiotics, cephalosporins, quinolones, and penicillins.

To ultrasound the kidney is incorrect. An appropriate diagnostic study should be ordered to exclude obstruction. In this young patient, without underlying reason for obstruction to occur, this is unlikely to be abnormal. Particularly in older men, both urinary catheterization for evidence of post-void residual and ultrasound are more likely to demonstrate evidence of obstructive uropathy.

A 24-hour urine for protein and creatinine clearance is incorrect. In the setting of acute renal failure, the creatinine clearance cannot be accurately determined as the creatinine is constantly rising, indicating that the patient must have markedly diminished GFR. In the absence of significant proteinuria, the 24-hour urine is unlikely to add further information in this patient.

A urine electrophoresis is not correct. This is the appropriate diagnostic study to order when one suspects light chains (Bence Jones protein) may be present in the urine. This is particularly important when evaluating patients for either multiple myeloma or amyloidosis. Amyloidosis is typically associated with nephrotic syndrome, which is not present in this patient, and amyloid of the kidney is usually also found when patients with myeloma also have nephrotic syndrome. A myeloma kidney may result in more tubular damage with little proteinuria; however, evidence of light chains in the urine may lead to the diagnosis.

An ANCA is not appropriate. Antineutrophilic cytoplasmic antibody is a useful diagnostic study in the evaluation of acute glomerulonephritis, particularly when either microscopic polyarteritis or Wegener's granulomatosis is suspected. This patient however has no significant hematuria or proteinuria, therefore making the diagnosis of acute glomerulonephritis most unlikely. While the ANCA may be very helpful in cases of rapidly progressive glomerulonephritis, it is not as helpful in the diagnosis of other forms of renal disease.

---

252. Answer: A

The correct answer is that the C-ANCA is likely to be positive. This patient has a "pulmonary-renal syndrome," and one should consider Goodpasture's syndrome, lupus, and Wegener's granulomatosis, though other causes are still possible. Whenever there is a rapidly progressive glomerulonephritis, regardless of etiology, one may see crescents in Bowman's space; however, lupus typically is associated with the presence of IgG, IgA, and IgM on immunofluorescent staining. Linear staining with IgG in the glomerular basement membrane is characteristic of Goodpasture's syndrome. While crescents are commonly found in patients with Wegener's granulomatosis, immunofluorescence is negative, but the C-ANCA will be positive in most patients. In a patient with features of chronic upper respiratory tract disease, pulmonary involvement, and glomerulonephritis, Wegener's granulomatosis is the most likely diagnosis and the C-ANCA is an important diagnostic tool.

The choice of P-ANCA will be positive is incorrect. The antineutrophil cytoplasmic antibody is an important diagnostic study in the evaluation of any patient with acute glomerulonephritis. P-ANCA (myeloperoxidase-MPO) is most likely to be positive in patients with microscopic polyarteritis, whereas C-ANCA (serine protease-PR3) will be positive most frequently in patients with Wegener's granulomatosis. While P-ANCA will be positive in many other forms of vasculitis, including systemic lupus, it will be the only serologic abnormality in patients with microscopic polyangiitis.

Based on the renal biopsy, initiating plasmapheresis is an incorrect choice. Plasmapheresis is the appropriate therapy in Goodpasture's syndrome. However, it is not appropriate in Wegener's where the standard therapy is corticosteroids and cyclophosphamide.

Significant eosinophilia is unlikely. Eosinophilia is an important clue in the diagnosis of Churg Strauss syndrome, not Wegener's. Those patients also present with asthma, an important clinical clue to the diagnosis of Churg Strauss.

Complement levels will not be low. In this patient without evidence of immune mediated glomerulonephritis, there is not likely to be complement activation, and complement levels are most likely to be normal.

---

253. Answer: D

The correct answer is this patient is not likely to develop progressive renal failure – the most likely diagnosis in the acute onset of severe nephrotic syndrome, particularly in a younger patient, is minimal change disease, which accounts for 10-15% of nephrotic syndrome in adults. The diagnosis is confirmed by renal biopsy and, in adults, the initial treatment is corticosteroid therapy. Most patients will respond to treatment with prednisone alone, though in adults, (as compared to pediatric minimal change disease), it is possible that cytotoxic therapy may need to be added to achieve remission. Patients who relapse after prednisone therapy should be retreated but frequent relapsers may also require cytotoxic therapy. In contrast to other types of glomerular disease, minimal change disease is not a progressive form of renal failure and the long-term prognosis is excellent.

It is incorrect to choose treatment that is initiated with steroids and cytotoxic therapy to prevent progressive renal disease. Initial therapy of adult minimal change disease is with prednisone alone with cytotoxic therapy being added only for patients who frequently relapse or in whom remission cannot be achieved.

An unlikely diagnosis is focal and segmental glomerulosclerosis. Focal and segmental glomerulosclerosis is an important cause of idiopathic nephrotic syndrome in adults and is the most common cause in African-Americans. FSGS presents with more insidious onset and is more commonly associated with both hypertension and impairment of renal function. Particularly in young African-American adults, presentation with idiopathic nephrotic syndrome, hypertension, and progressive renal failure strongly suggests the diagnosis of FSGS. FSGS is also treated with prednisone initially, with those patients achieving remission having a significantly better prognosis.

Another incorrect choice would be treatment initiated with cyclosporine – while cyclosporin has been used for treatment of steroid resistant minimal change disease in children, it is not considered initial therapy in either adults or children. It has been used in some trials in both steroid resistant minimal change disease and steroid resistant focal segmental glomerulosclerosis with variable degrees of success.

Finally, ACE inhibitor therapy should be used in patients with heavy proteinuria. ACE inhibitors exert an important anti-proteinuric affect and should be used in patients with hypertension and proteinuria. However, they may also be an important adjunct to therapy in patients with heavy proteinuria even with normotension.

---

254. Answer: C

The correct answer is to order complement levels. The presence of RBC casts establishes the diagnosis of glomerulonephritis, therefore complete serologic studies to exclude secondary causes is essential. The most likely diagnosis in a patient with gross hematuria immediately following an upper respiratory infection is IgA nephropathy. While the diagnosis can only be established by renal biopsy, complement levels and hepatitis studies must be performed to exclude underlying secondary causes, such as lupus, post-infectious glomerulonephritis, or HCV-associated GN.

Referral to urologist is incorrect. It is essential to determine in patients with hematuria whether the bleeding is most likely coming from the upper or lower tract. Clues to the diagnosis of upper tract bleeding include the presence of red blood cell casts, proteinuria associated with hematuria, and dysmorphic red blood cells. In patients with isolated hematuria where none of these features are present, urologic evaluation would be appropriate, particularly in older patients where the diagnosis of GU malignancy must be excluded. This patient has glomerulonephritis based on the RBC casts and urologic referral would only delay diagnosis.

Immediate referral for renal biopsy is incorrect. Patients who present with evidence of glomerulonephritis will usually require renal biopsy to establish a diagnosis. Of particular concern are those patients with acute glomerulonephritis as manifested by evidence of salt and water retention with renal insufficiency. Patients with rapidly progressive glomerulonephritis in which renal function can deteriorate even on a daily basis should always be evaluated for urgent renal biopsy to quickly establish a diagnosis and initiate appropriate therapy. In this patient, outpatient evaluation should be performed before biopsy is performed.

It is incorrect to begin prednisone 60 mg daily. Patients with IgA nephropathy and normal renal function, especially without proteinuria, require no therapy. Of greater concern are patients with progressive disease who are likely to have significant proteinuria. More recent studies have evaluated the use of both steroid and cytotoxic therapy in patients with proteinuria and progressive renal disease with data suggesting these treatments may be of benefit. This would not be appropriate in this patient.

Hearing evaluation is not indicated. One of the considerations in younger patients who present with hematuria due to glomerulonephritis is Alport's syndrome (hereditary nephritis). The hallmarks of this disorder are hearing loss and glomerulonephritis, occasionally with associated ocular abnormalities. This disease is typically expressed much more severely in men than in women. While the family history can be very suggestive, the diagnosis can only be established with certainty by renal biopsy demonstrating particular thinning or lamellation of the glomerular basement membrane seen on electron microscopy.

---

255. Answer: E

The correct answer is to administer calcium gluconate. This patient has acute renal failure secondary to rhabdomyolysis, and has developed a bradyarrhythmia secondary to hyperkalemia. The clinical presentation and the markedly elevated CPK are adequate to establish the diagnosis, even before the urine myoglobin is available. It is important to realize that this test may be negative depending on when it is obtained. The presence of 4+ blood without red blood cells on microscopic examination associated with granular casts is characteristic of ATN associated with rhabdomyolysis. In patients who become oliguric, particularly with severe muscle injury, hyperkalemia can be a potentially lethal complication. Initially T waves may become peaked, but as hyperkalemia worsens, patients may develop variable degrees of heart block, eventually resulting in third-degree heart block and severe conduction delays. Such patients are at risk of cardiac arrest. The first step in the emergency treatment of hyperkalemia is to administer calcium to stabilize the cardiac membrane. This can be administered as 10 ml of 10% calcium gluconate over ten minutes, followed by glucose and insulin, which will then push potassium back into the cells until the total potassium burden can be removed through dialysis or other therapy.

It is incorrect to administer Kayexalate enemas. Kayexalate is inappropriate for the emergency therapy of hyperkalemia. The onset of action is several hours and Kayexalate should only be used in life-threatening hyperkalemia after treatment with calcium, glucose, and insulin or other agents have been administered, particularly if dialysis is not available.

Initiate dialysis therapy is not correct. Hyperkalemia and acute renal failure are clearly an indication for dialysis; however, medical therapy should always be the initial therapy while awaiting dialysis, and in patients with EKG changes, calcium should be administered. It would be appropriate to obtain urgent consultation in such a patient but it would be incumbent on the treating physicians to manage the patient medically until dialysis could be initiated.

Temporary pacemaker placement is not indicated. Recognition of this patient's heart block as being due to hyperkalemia is essential in the appropriate management. In the setting of rhabdomyolysis and acute renal failure, the diagnosis of hyperkalemia as the cause of heart block must be considered and therefore the heart block will resolve once hyperkalemia is appropriately treated. Even in patients who demonstrate hemodynamic instability, immediate treatment of hyperkalemia typically resolves heart block and therefore pacing is usually not necessary.

To perform fasciotomies is incorrect. While fasciotomy may be necessary in patients with compartment syndromes and persistent rhabdomyolysis, this would not be appropriate initial therapy with life-threatening arrhythmia secondary to hyperkalemia.

256. Answer: C

The correct answer is metabolic acidosis, respiratory alkalosis, and metabolic alkalosis. While it is apparent that this patient has diabetic ketoacidosis, it may not be apparent that she has a triple acid base disorder. In evaluating all patients with electrolyte and acid base disorders, the anion gap must also be calculated. In this patient, the anion gap is 32, which is consistent with her anion gap metabolic acidosis associated with diabetic ketoacidosis. When one calculates what the PCO_2 should be for a patient with metabolic acidosis with a serum bicarbonate of 12 (1.5 x HCO3 + 8), that value is 26. This patient's PCO_2 is 20 so she is therefore overventilating and therefore must also have a respiratory alkalosis. Finally one can also calculate the "delta anion gap," which is the amount of bicarbonate that has been consumed to raise the anion gap from the normal value of 12 to 32 in this patient, which is 20. Since the patient consumed 20 millimoles of bicarbonate per liter and her current serum bicarbonate is 12 then she must have had an "initial" bicarbonate of 32 (20 + 12 = 32). This therefore uncovers the hidden metabolic alkalosis, which one would expect in a patient with severe vomiting. Appropriate therapy is still fluid resuscitation and insulin administration, while watching for the development of hypokalemia.

257. Answer: E

The correct answer is Bartter's syndrome. In evaluating metabolic alkalosis, it is extremely helpful to order urine chloride, which will be elevated when the alkalosis is due to both endogenous and exogenous steroid excess or due to Bartter's syndrome. Bartter's syndrome is caused by a mutation of the Na-K 2-chloride transporter in the thick ascending limb of Henle. Bartter's syndrome is a familial disorder characterized by metabolic alkalosis, normotension, normokalemia, hypomagnesemia, and elevated renin and aldosterone levels.

Liddle's syndrome is incorrect. This familial disorder is characterized by hypertension, hypokalemia, and low renin and aldosterone. It is caused by a defect in the collecting duct sodium channel. Amiloride is the appropriate treatment.

Primary hyperaldosteronism is incorrect. These patients present with hypertension, hypokalemia, and metabolic alkalosis. Renin levels are low while aldosterone levels are high and non-suppressible. Primary hyperaldosteronism is due to either unilateral adrenal adenoma or bilateral adrenal hyperplasia.

Addison's disease is incorrect. Patients with Addison's disease have mineralocorticoid deficiency and therefore are normotensive or hypotensive with hyperkalemia and a metabolic acidosis.

Renal artery stenosis is incorrect. Patients with renal artery stenosis may be hypokalemic with a metabolic alkalosis, but they are hypertensive. These patients have secondary hyperaldosteronism and therefore renin levels are also elevated.

258. Answer: B

The correct answer is an ACE inhibitor. Clinical studies clearly show that ACE inhibitors may slow the progression of renal disease in patients with diabetes and therefore they should be considered first-line therapy for the treatment of hypertension. All diabetics should be screened with protein:creatinine ratios on a yearly basis, which can be done using either a random urine specimen sent to the lab for protein and creatinine determinations with a ratio of greater than 30mg/g constituting microalbuminuria. This corresponds with a 24-hour urine collection of between 30-200 mg of protein per day. In either normotensive diabetics with a protein to creatinine ratio of greater than 30 or hypertensive diabetics, therapy should be initiated with ACE inhibitors, though ARBs are also acceptable as initial therapy. It is essential that one check the serum potassium to make sure the patient doesn't have an underlying Type IV renal tubular acidosis with subsequent hyperkalemia prior to initiating one of these agents.

A thiazide diuretic is incorrect. While diabetics particularly with renal disease may have evidence of volume retention and an expanded extracellular fluid volume contributing to their hypertension, diuretics should be added after ACE inhibitor therapy. Diuretics are also particularly helpful in African-Americans because the addition of a diuretic to an ACE inhibitor may enhance efficacy of action.

Minoxidil is incorrect. Minoxidil is a very potent vasodilator that is effective in the treatment of refractory hypertension and may therefore be useful in the management of diabetics with particularly difficult-to-control hypertension. It may however cause fluid retention, reflex tachycardia, and hirsutism and is not initial therapy.

Nifedipine is incorrect. While there is some evidence that calcium channel blockers may reduce proteinuria in hypertensive diabetics with proteinuria, the data is more strongly associated with diltiazem than the dihydropyridine calcium channel blockers. These agents therefore should not be used in initial therapy in diabetics, and if a calcium channel blocker is used, it may be more appropriate to use diltiazem.

A beta-blocker is an incorrect choice. Particularly for diabetics who have had myocardial infarction, beta-blockers should certainly be given; however, they should not be used as initial therapy if there is no contraindication to the use of an ACE inhibitor.

---

259. Answer: B

The correct answer is Type I distal RTA. This patient has a non-anion gap (NAG) metabolic acidosis. The initial approach in NAG metabolic acidosis is to measure the urinary anion gap. This serves as a measure of urinary acidification. Normally the urine anion gap (Urine Na + K – Cl) is negative. However in patients with urinary acidification defects, this value will be positive. Normally one should be able to acidify the urine in the face of metabolic acidosis. In this patient, the urine pH is 7 because he cannot secrete H+ ions across the concentration gradient in the distal tubule. These patients cannot lower their urine pH below 6.0 regardless of degree of acidosis. These patients also have hypercalciuria, and may develop nephrolithiasis and nephrocalcinosis. Congenital, familial RTA is associated with hearing loss, while acquired Type I RTA is seen with several underlying disorders, including hyperparathyroidism and hypergammaglobulinemia. Treatment includes bicarbonate and potassium administration.

Type II RTA is incorrect. These patients typically "waste" bicarbonate, and therefore the urine pH is also high initially, along with a NAG metabolic acidosis. Eventually patients have no more $HC0_3$ to waste and the urine pH becomes more acid. Proximal RTA may also be associated with Fanconi syndrome and urinary loss of glucose, phosphorus, uric acid, and amino acids. This disorder is not associated with nephrolithiasis or hearing loss. Important causes of acquired Type II RTA include multiple myeloma and heavy metals. These patients may require large amounts of bicarbonate administration to correct the acidosis.

Type IV RTA is incorrect. Type IV RTA is a hyperkalemic distal RTA, most commonly occurring in diabetics, but also associated with obstructive uropathy and other forms of tubulointerstitial renal disease. It is most often caused by aldosterone deficiency. Treatment includes sodium bicarbonate administration, fludrocortisone, and/or furosemide.

Chronic diarrhea is not a correct choice. Chronic diarrhea and HCO_3 loss may cause a NAG metabolic acidosis. However, urinary acidification is normal, therefore the urinary anion gap will be negative.

Salicylate intoxication is not likely. Salicylate intoxication causes an anion gap metabolic acidosis and is not associated with hypokalemia. Patients typically also have a respiratory alkalosis, which serves as another clue to the diagnosis.

---

260. Answer: D

The correct answer is impaired renal excretion due to Type IV renal tubular acidosis. Diabetes is the most common cause of Type IV renal tubular acidosis, presenting with Type II DM and mild renal insufficiency. The urinary symptoms also suggest that he has prostatic hypertrophy and possible mild chronic urinary tract obstruction, another common cause of Type IV renal tubular acidosis. Acidosis can cause movement of potassium out of cells usually in the setting of metabolic acidosis. The degree of hyperkalemia is out of proportion to his degree of acidemia and his acidosis is predominantly a respiratory acidosis. Likewise, his degree of hyperkalemia is out of proportion to his degree of renal failure. Renal handling of potassium is maintained generally until glomerular filtration falls below 15 to 20 ml/min. Pseudohyperkalemia is unlikely in view of the EKG findings. Excessive dietary potassium intake is an extraordinarily rare cause of hyperkalemia.

---

261. Answer: E

The correct answer is begin hydrochlorothiazide 25 mg/day. This patient most likely has congenital nephrogenic diabetes insipidus. He has thirst and polyuria. His serum sodium is borderline, elevated with a relatively low urine osmolality. Neither serum nor urine suggests diabetes mellitus as a cause of his polyuria. He had a childhood history of enuresis and has never presented for medical attention. Most patients with nephrogenic diabetes insipidus learn to live with their polyuria and do not consider themselves "ill." The only treatment for nephrogenic diabetes insipidus of unknown etiology is hydrochlorothiazide as thiazide diuretics enhance distal tubule water reabsorption. The lifelong history of polyuria and the ability to concentrate the urine to near 300 mOsm/kg suggests that he does not have central diabetes insipidus, so neither vasopressin tannate in oil nor DDAVP would be effective. Water restriction would result in further hypernatremia. Although it may stimulate his kidneys to concentrate his urine somewhat more than they presently are, it would not be adequate to maintain a reasonable serum osmolality. The patient's relative hypernatremia argues strongly against a diagnosis of psychogenic polydipsia.

---

262. Answer: A

The correct answer is dipsticks only detect negatively charged proteins like albumin. Immunoglobulins (which is likely what he is excreting) are positively charged and therefore are not picked up on the dipstick.

---

263. Answer: C

The correct answer is nephrogenic diabetes insipidus. Failure to concentrate urine in the face of substantial hypertonic dehydration suggests diabetes insipidus. A nephrogenic origin is suspected when there is no increase in urine concentration after exogenous vasopressin.

264. Answer: D

The correct answer is Na 143, K 4.8, Cl-100, HCO_3-10, Serum Creatinine 3.5, and Arterial pH 7.25. Ethylene glycol ingestion causes acute renal failure and leads to rapid accumulation of metabolic acids. Acidosis is proportionate to the degree of renal insufficiency and is characterized by a HIGH anion gap (here, AG = 33).

265. Answer: B

The correct answer is Na 140, K 2.6, Cl-115, HCO_3-13, Serum Creatinine 3.5, Arterial pH 7.31, and urine pH 6.2. Amphotericin B also causes renal insufficiency with a disproportionate metabolic acidosis. However, the acidosis is due to a distal tubular acidification defect and is characterized by hyperchloremia, a normal anion gap, and inability to lower the urine pH.

266. Answer: A

The correct answer is Na 136, K 5.2, Cl-102, HCO_3-20, Serum Creatinine 3.5, Arterial pH 7.36, and urine pH 5.0. With a moderate glomerulonephritis, metabolic acidosis is usually mild and the anion gap is only slightly if at all elevated.

267. Answer: E

The correct answer is Na 140, K 6.2, Cl-109, HCO_3-20, Serum Creatinine 3.5, Arterial pH 7.36, and urine pH 5.0. This illustrates moderate renal insufficiency with disproportionate hyperkalemia and hyperchloremic acidosis. One of the most common things to do this is diabetic nephropathy.

268. Answer: D

The correct answer is Na 135, K 4.5, Cl-106, HCO_3-22, Serum Creatinine 3.5, Arterial pH 7.37, and urine pH 5.0. This answer illustrates a decrease in the anion gap, which is most frequently reported with multiple myeloma. The apparent reduction is due to a circulating paraprotein that bears a positive charge.

269. Answer: C

The correct answer is selective elevation of LDL cholesterol with increased atherogenesis. The risk of myositis is increased but not by very much. HMG-CoA reductase inhibitors work well, but should not be combined with fibric acid derivatives.

270. Answer: B

The correct answer is Check TSH; this is an unusual presentation of hypothyroidism. This patient has signs and symptoms of hypothyroidism and the next test that should be ordered is a TSH level, which is expected to be markedly increased. The obvious evidence for hypothyroidism includes feeling tired, moving slowly, talking slowly, and dry skin. But don't overlook the galactorrhea, pituitary mass, and mildly elevated prolactin level. At first glance, this can be mistaken for a prolactinoma, but a prolactinoma of this size (macroadenoma) should be associated with prolactin levels > 200 ng/mL. A prolactin level < 100 ng/mL should always prompt you to look elsewhere, in this case the thyroid. Some other causes of a mildly elevated prolactin that have been ruled out include pregnancy and excessive nipple stimulation. The pituitary mass in this patient is most likely not a tumor. It is a pseudotumor comprised of TSH-secreting cells (thyrotrophs), which have hypertrophied in response to TRH stimulation. TRH also stimulates the secretion of prolactin, hence the elevated levels.

It would be inappropriate to treat with bromocriptine or surgery. There is no reason to look for a non-pituitary cancer. Re-checking the prolactin level would be appropriate at some time in the future, but her hypothyroidism must be addressed first.

---

271. Answer: D

The correct answer is switch him to cabergoline (Dostinex). The question states that the patient has a prolactinoma and is being treated with bromocriptine. Unfortunately, he is experiencing considerable nausea and vomiting, which are common side effects of bromocriptine and many patients are unable to tolerate it. An alternative drug, cabergoline, is available. This drug is just as effective at reducing prolactin levels and is much less likely to cause nausea and vomiting. Unfortunately, cabergoline is expensive. Bromocriptine is the usual drug of choice with cabergoline usually held in reserve.

It would be inappropriate to just stop the bromocriptine without starting cabergoline because he would most likely experience a flare-up in his symptoms. Resection of a prolactinoma should only be done when the mass effects of a large tumor warrant it, such as an impaired field of vision or seizures. Adding Compazine for nausea is not appropriate because he hasn't tried a course of cabergoline. Finally, the addition of cabergoline to bromocriptine should not be done. These two drugs work the same way and using them together would not be expected to lessen the severity of the nausea and vomiting.

---

272. Answer: E

The correct answer is start bromocriptine and repeat the CT/MRI in a few days. This patient has a large prolactinoma and the primary physician wants it to be removed. However, in the absence of visual field defects, seizures, severe headaches, etc., the surgery is not emergent and can probably wait a few days. In the meantime, start the patient on bromocriptine. This drug will shrink the tumor and may shrink it enough to avoid surgery. Though it usually takes much more than a few days to show an appreciable reduction in size, the prolactinoma may nevertheless begin to shrink within a short period of time. Beginning the pre-operative evaluation is justified, but it is more important to begin bromocriptine. High-dose glucocorticoids may be justified if symptomatic, but are not needed in this case.

---

273. Answer: E

The correct answer is check serum IGF-1 and 24-hour urine cortisol. Whenever a pituitary incidentaloma is discovered, two main questions must be answered. One, is the mass inhibiting secretion of any pituitary tumors. Two, is the tumor secreting something. Let's review the inhibiting scenario first. Many pituitary tumors do not appear to secrete anything and are called null cell tumors. With the advent of sensitive assays, it has been learned that some of these null-cell tumors actually do secrete. They may be secreting α-chains or gonadotrophins (LH or FSH), which rarely cause symptoms. After all, which man is going to complain about larger testes or a higher sperm count. However, some of these tumors get large enough that they inhibit secretion of pituitary hormones because of a mass effect. In this patient, the tumor is a microadenoma (< 10 mm) and is too small to inhibit secretion.

The other scenario is one of excess secretion. Does the pituitary tumor secrete any hormones? Remember the main 6 anterior pituitary hormones: ACTH, LH, FSH, GH, TSH, and PRL. A fishing expedition to test all hormones is not recommended. Instead, evaluate the patient for signs or symptoms that may point toward a particular excess such as galactorrhea or loss of libido (PRL); amenorrhea (LH, FSH); weight loss, hyperdefecation, tachyarrhythmia, heat intolerance (TSH); hypertension, hypokalemia, alkalosis (ACTH). These findings can be very subtle or even absent in the case of a new tumor or a very small one. If your evaluation does not point toward a particular hormone, then check the adrenal and thyroid axes. A screening test for the adrenal axis is a 24-hour urine for cortisol and a value < 70 µg is normal. The thyroid axis can be checked by a TSH and T4 drawn at any time of the day.

I must caution you to check one more hormone. A small tumor may be secreting GH. The effects of over-secretion of GH takes many years to become evident and many more years usually transpire before it is recognized. These patients develop acromegaly and its many serious complications. Though GH is pulsatile, its effect on IGF-1 is not. Measure a random IGF-1 in any patient with a pituitary incidentaloma. In this patient, the central obesity and hypertension may indicate hypercortisolism (Cushing's syndrome). Order a 24-hour urine for cortisol and don't forget to check the IGF-1 level.

"Refer him to a neurosurgeon for transsphenoidal resection of the pituitary mass" is incorrect because there are no reasons to refer this patient for surgery at this time.

"Return to your clinic in a few weeks to recheck blood pressure" is incorrect because the pituitary tumor must be evaluated and his blood pressure management must be followed.

"Discharge him from your clinic on a drug to treat hypertension and encourage him to stop riding motorcycles" is incorrect because, once again, the pituitary tumor must be evaluated.

"Check an ACTH stimulation test, TSH, and a total testosterone" is incorrect because hyposecretion of ACTH, secondary hypothyroidism, and secondary hypogonadism are not suspected.

---

274. Answer: A

The correct answer is: Tell her that everything is normal and discharge her from your clinic. The important point to remember for this question is that an empty sella may be normal. This patient does not present any indication of pituitary dysfunction. The history of blood loss at the time of delivery may suggest Sheehan's syndrome (hemorrhagic necrosis of the pituitary), but one of the most sensitive indicators of pituitary dysfunction is ovulation. This patient was able to get pregnant six more times; the hypothalamic-pituitary-ovarian axis must be working properly. She does not have Sheehan's syndrome, but her obstetrical history offers another clue. Her seven pregnancies have most likely caused her empty sella. With pregnancy, the pituitary enlarges and has a greater blood flow. This produces an upward pressure on the diaphragm covering the top of the sella, which stretches and expands the diaphragm. After pregnancy, the pituitary returns to a normal size with a normal blood flow, but the diaphragm is acellular and remains stretched. With each subsequent pregnancy, the diaphragm becomes progressively more stretched. This allows the diaphragm to bulge downward and into the sella under the pressure of the CSF fluid above it. In some cases, the diaphragm has become so loose that the CSF fluid displaces the majority of the pituitary to the periphery of the sella. A CT of the head will fail to identify pituitary tissue and the term "empty sella" will be used. In actuality, the sella is not empty, but contains CSF fluid and normal pituitary tissue that has been pushed to the periphery. The pituitary tissue can work perfectly normal in this environment.

It is inappropriate to refer her to a neurosurgeon. Pituitary exploration may disrupt the normal functioning of her existing pituitary tissue and result in the development of hypopituitarism. While there is no evidence of pituitary dysfunction, the abdominal striae may trick some people to suspect Cushing's syndrome, but there is no mention of hyperglycemia, hypokalemia, or the typical body habitus. Stretch marks are a common occurrence, especially following pregnancy. The typical stretch marks associated with Cushing's syndrome are broad and appear purplish from the coloration of underlying tissue.

275. Answer: C

The correct answer is Check FT4 and TSH. Many things can cause an unexplained weight loss, and depression is common in elderly patients. However, these symptoms are also associated with hyperthyroidism. Unfortunately, elderly individuals do not always exhibit the adrenergic response to hyperthyroidism. The term apathetic hyperthyroidism refers to hyperthyroidism without the usual manifestations of tremor, palpitations, heat intolerance, etc. The only sign exhibited by the patient in this question is tachycardia.

Unexplained weight loss with a long history of smoking should always make you suspicious of cancer. Most physicians would order a chest x-ray. When it comes back normal, one should rethink the case. The thyroid should be evaluated before more extensive screening for cancer takes place. Depression is common and it may be appropriate either to begin treating him or to refer him to a psychiatrist. However, do not forget that hyperthyroidism can cause depression. If the patient has hyperthyroidism and depression, it is not appropriate to treat the depression while ignoring the hyperthyroidism. Treat the hyperthyroidism and follow the depression; the depression will often resolve once the patient is euthyroid. Finally, one should always encourage proper eating habits and appropriate exercise.

276. Answer: B

The correct answer is counsel her on her risk of having an MI and begin low-dose thyroxine therapy. This patient is euthyroid and appears healthy. Should she just come back to see you in one year or should you be more aggressive? The Rotterdam study (Hak AE, *et al.* Ann Intern Med. 2000;132:270-8) showed that a woman > 55 years old with a TSH > 4 μIU/mL has an increased risk of experiencing an MI. You should inform her of this risk. The issue of treatment in this situation is not clear-cut. Large prospective studies showing a reduction in MI with treatment in this scenario have not yet been reported, but small studies suggest a possible benefit with low-dose thyroxine. The issues should be reviewed with the patient so that she can make an informed decision. However, low-dose thyroxine is generally benign and its use in this scenario may be warranted. The treatment goal is to lower the TSH to within the range of 1-4 μIU/mL. Another possible benefit from treating her subclinical hypothyroidism may be a decline in her cholesterol level.

Simply telling her that everything is fine may seem acceptable, but the better course of action is to discuss the issue with her and to suggest thyroxine. In the absence of symptoms (polyuria and polydipsia) and a low index of suspicion, her glucose does not need to be repeated again for at least one year. There is no indication for a repeat pelvic examination by a gynecologist. According to the National Cholesterol Education Program (NCEP) guidelines, she does not need to be started on statins at this time. Moreover, her liver function tests must be checked before initiating statin therapy.

277. Answer: D

The correct answer is begin thyroxine 25 μg PO QD and follow her heart condition closely. This patient has severe hypothyroidism along with poor cardiac function. Though hypothyroidism impairs cardiac function, it also decreases the demand being placed on the heart. Thus the heart is not always working as hard in hypothyroidism as it may be working in someone who is euthyroid. There is no question that her hypothyroidism needs to be addressed, but you are being asked to choose which treatment is most appropriate. Intravenous thyroxine will rapidly correct her hypothyroidism, especially with the addition of triiodothyronine, but this will also rapidly increase the demands placed on her heart. In the face of her impaired cardiac function, this sudden increased demand could easily exceed her cardiac capacity and have dire consequences. The remaining three choices are all oral thyroxine at different strengths. The most appropriate choice in this case is the 25 μg dose. This dose will not have much effect on her hypothyroidism, so it will not greatly increase her cardiac work. The dose can be steadily increased every few months if she tolerates it. The best course of action is to start low and go slow. This will give her heart a chance to increase its conditioning and to be able to tolerate the next dose increase.

278. Answer: C

The correct answer is the patient probably does not have any thyroid problems. This patient is critically sick. In severe illness, the pituitary secretes less TSH, which results in a low or low-normal FT4. However, T4 is not the active hormone; T3 is active. In severe illness, T3 levels are greatly suppressed. With the T4 being lower, there is less T4 available to be converted into T3. However, there is still considerable T4 present. In order to protect the body from the active T3 hormone, the T4 is converted into an inactive hormone call reverse T3 (rT3). Levels of rT3 are rarely measured, but if it was measured in this patient, it would be greatly elevated.

This patient is most likely euthyroid, but very sick. He does not have hypothyroidism or hyperthyroidism, either primary or secondary. There is no need to treat his abnormal thyroid tests other than to treat his underlying illness.

279. Answer: B

The correct answer is refer him for a thyroid fine-needle biopsy and aspiration (FNA). This patient is euthyroid, but with a thyroid nodule. The correct answer is to perform a thyroid FNA, either yourself or refer him to someone who can. If the biopsy is not conclusive, then repeat it. If the second biopsy is also inconclusive, then refer him to a surgeon for a hemithyroidectomy. A near-total thyroidectomy would only be needed if cancer was present. Many physicians in the past have tried to shrink nodules with thyroxine, thinking that exogenous thyroxine will lower the TSH, which will reduce the growth stimulation to the nodule. Unfortunately, studies have shown this not to be the case; thyroxine should not be given in the hope of shrinking a nodule. Considering how easy and safe a thyroid biopsy is, it would be inappropriate to just follow him. Though the vast majority of nodules are benign, cancer cannot be excluded by simply watching the nodule.

280. Answer: A

The correct answer is begin anti-thyroid medication now and postpone the surgery until he is euthyroid or nearly so. This question requires you to understand the dangers of hyperthyroidism in a patient going into surgery. This patient has signs of hyperthyroidism, which is verified by laboratory tests. In a patient with hyperthyroidism, any kind of surgery can trigger a severe uncompensated hyperthyroidism (thyroid storm), which can be fatal. Treatment of the hyperthyroidism should be initiated before the surgery takes place. The question of whether to postpone the operation is a little more problematic and depends on whether the surgery is emergent, urgent, or routine. Obviously, if the surgery is an emergency and cannot be postponed, ask the anesthesiologist to administer iodine to inhibit thyroid hormone synthesis (this can be administered as intravenous radiocontrast agents), β-blockers to block the adrenergic effects of hyperthyroidism, and glucocorticoids to protect from the stress of hyperthyroidism and to inhibit the conversion of T4 to T3. If the surgery is routine and can be delayed, as in this case, the patient should be started on anti-thyroid medications and the operation should be postponed until the patient is rendered euthyroid or nearly euthyroid. An operation that is urgent, but not emergent, can be postponed for a limited amount of time. During this interval, begin anti-thyroid medications (PTU or methimazole), iodide, and β-blockers. Though the patient will probably not be euthyroid before surgery, his hyperthyroidism will at least be lessened in severity and may protect him from developing thyroid storm.

281. Answer: D

The correct answer is order TSH and FT4, suspecting hypothyroidism due to postpartum thyroiditis. Many young mothers will report postpartum depression, which will resolve on its own. However, some of these cases of postpartum depression may actually signify postpartum thyroiditis. The typical presentation is an uneventful pregnancy and delivery followed by an initial period of hyperthyroidism lasting for about one month, which is followed by a protracted period of hypothyroidism lasting for many months and sometimes for a year. The initial period of hyperthyroidism is easily tolerated. After all, the woman will have considerable energy and will lose weight more easily. However, she will soon develop hypothyroidism. Once you verify with TSH and FT4 that she is hypothyroid, begin treating her with thyroxine. Her hyperthyroidism is not likely to be permanent, so follow her monthly and adjust the thyroxine dose as needed, ultimately discontinuing it.

282. Answer: B

The correct answer is he has diabetes and must talk with a diabetes educator and dietitian to begin a diet and exercise program. He fulfills two diagnostic criteria for the diagnosis of diabetes. The full set of criteria include (1) random glucose ≥ 200 mg/dL with symptoms (polyuria, polydipsia, or unexplained weight loss), (2) fasting glucose ≥ 126 mg/dL, and (3) 2-hour 75 g oral glucose tolerance test (OGTT) ≥ 200 mg/dL. Now that you have diagnosed him with diabetes, you must next determine whether he has type 1 or type 2 diabetes. He most likely has type 2 because he is overweight and there is no mention of metabolic decompensation. You must now determine whether to treat and, if so, how to treat his diabetes. There is no question about it; you must intervene immediately. There is nothing to benefit from waiting. However, in the absence of metabolic decompensation and severe hyperglycemia, it is most prudent to begin with lifestyle changes. He must be educated on the importance of an exercise program (walking is usually enough) and he must learn how to eat a healthy diet. Diet and exercise may be all that he needs. Only if he fails such a regimen should he be started on drug therapy.

283. Answer: E

The correct answer is stop taking the metformin and to come to your office tomorrow. It is important to know the contraindications for use of metformin. Of course it is absolutely contraindicated when the patient has a known hypersensitivity to it or any component of the pill, but also in men with a creatinine ≥ 1.5 mg/dL or in women with a creatinine ≥ 1.4 mg/dL. This is a very commonly used drug and these numbers must be memorized for proper patient care. It is not unreasonable to be expected to know these numbers on an examination. It is also important to know that relative contraindications include kidney, liver, and heart dysfunction.

He has good glycemic control and does not need a second agent at this time. There is no compelling reason to add a thiazolidinedione. The recommended LDL goal in a diabetic is < 100 mg/dL. His LDL is currently at goal and does not need a statin drug. In light of his creatinine level of 1.5 mg/dL, it is inappropriate to simply have him return to your clinic in 6 months. The blood pressure goal for a diabetic without albuminuria is < 130/80. His blood pressure is not elevated and he does not need to start any blood pressure-lowering agents at this time.

284. Answer: B

The correct answer is to reduce drastically her evening NPH insulin and to decrease the evening insulin even further if the symptoms do not improve. Her symptoms of vivid nightmares and waking in a cold sweat are compatible with nocturnal hypoglycemia. The most likely explanation for the early morning hyperglycemia is that the nocturnal hypoglycemia is causing the contrainsular hormones (glucagon, cortisol, growth hormone, and epinephrine) to be secreted. Many type 1 diabetics lose the ability to secrete glucagon in response to hypoglycemia, but the remaining hormones are unaffected. These hormones will raise the glucose level. However, insulin-deficient persons such as this patient do not have the ability to make their own insulin to control the hyperglycemic effect of the contrainsular hormones, and her morning fasting glucose levels are elevated. Every patient taking insulin needs to perform self-monitoring of their blood glucose levels. They should check their glucose before and two hours after every meal, at bedtime, and in the middle of the night around 3 a.m. Of course it's impractical to constantly check glucose levels this often on a daily basis. One alternative is to have patients check their glucose level twice every day, choosing different times each day so that the log book will have some numbers at each time point. The 3 a.m. glucose level should be checked at least once each month, but doesn't need to be checked much more frequently unless the patient is having evidence of nocturnal hypoglycemia or has changed the insulin regimen. Once this patient no longer has hypoglycemia, the insulin can always be carefully and slowly increased.

It is inappropriate to begin an anxiolytic rather than decreasing the insulin. Hypoglycemia can be life threatening. Increasing her evening insulin further could be fatal. There is no evidence that she has insulin resistance in addition to her insulin deficiency and adding an insulin sensitizer is inappropriate. Switching her to a 70/30 premix is also inappropriate. The goal of treating a type 1 diabetic is to replace the insulin in a physiologic way. Her insulin regimen is already physiologic by offering basal coverage with NPH twice daily and bolus coverage with a rapid-acting insulin analog with each meal.

---

285. Answer: C

The correct answer is add an ACE inhibitor or an angiotensin receptor blocker (ARB).

The random urine screen indicates microalbuminuria. Normal albumin excretion is < 30 mg/day, microalbuminuria is 30-300 mg/day, and macroalbuminuria is > 300 mg/day. Collecting an accurate 24-hour urine is difficult and problematic. Fortunately, creatinine excretion is somewhat consistent when adjusted for standard body surface area. This has led to use of the albumin:creatinine ratio in a random spot urine as a surrogate marker. A normal ratio is < 30 µg/mg, microalbuminuria is 30-300 µg/mg, and macroalbuminuria is > 300 µg/mg. If the ratio is only slightly above normal, it is best to repeat the random urine or to ask for a 24-hour urine to better quantitate the albumin excretion. In addition, any urinary tract infection must be completely resolved before checking for albuminuria. His ratio is well within the range of microalbuminuria and there is no suspicion of a urinary tract infection. Once a diabetic has microalbuminuria, the patient must be treated. The goal of treatment is to slow the progression of the nephropathy in an attempt to prevent end-stage renal disease. Several studies have shown that an ACE inhibitor is an excellent drug for this purpose and some recent studies have shown that angiotensin receptor blockers (ARB) may be just as beneficial. The best course of action for this patient is to begin one of these drugs.

The patient is certainly doing a good job by watching his diet, consistently walking, and losing weight. He should be praised for this, but he also needs treatment for the nephropathy. There is no reason to increase his statin since the LDL is less than 100 mg/dL (goal). A calcium channel blocker may be useful for hypertension, but is not the initial drug of choice in diabetics with nephropathy. Likewise, a diuretic can be useful for blood pressure control, but is not the initial drug of choice in a diabetic with nephropathy.

---

286. Answer: D

The correct diagnosis is primary hyperparathyroidism. The PTH is elevated along with the calcium. Normally, an elevated calcium would suppress the PTH level. His PTH is elevated in the face of hypercalcemia and thus represents primary hyperparathyroidism.

His vitamin D levels are elevated, but this is due to both his primary hyperparathyroidism and his use of vitamin supplements. Vitamin A intoxication can cause hypercalcemia, but no vitamin A levels are given in this question and his primary hyperparathyroidism is a better explanation. Pseudopseudohypoparathyroidism refers to a specific phenotype (shortened 4th and 5th metacarpals) with normal calcium and parathyroid hormone levels. His labs rule out such a diagnosis. Secondary hyperparathyroidism refers to the normally elevated levels of parathyroid hormone in the face of hypocalcemia. Low calcium levels will stimulate the parathyroid glands to secrete extra hormone, which will stimulate the conversion of 25OH-vitamin D into 1,25$(OH)_2$-vitamin D. His calcium is elevated and thus cannot have secondary hyperparathyroidism.

287. Answer: B

The correct answer is Vitamin D deficiency. This lady has probably had hypocalcemia for quite some time and only came to medical attention because she experienced an osteoporotic hip fracture. An extremely common cause of hypocalcemia is vitamin D deficiency and she exhibits a classic presentation. Her 25OH-Vitamin D level is low, reflecting both her poor diet and her low exposure to sunlight due to her reluctance to leave the house. Hypocalcemia normally gives rise to an elevated parathyroid hormone level (secondary hyperparathyroidism) and this in turn stimulates the conversion of 25OH-Vitamin D to 1,25$(OH)_2$-Vitamin D. Unfortunately, her levels of 25OH-Vitamin D are already low and her conversion to 1,25$(OH)_2$-Vitamin D is thus impaired. The phosphate level is low because of the hyperparathyroidism, which stimulates renal excretion of phosphates.

While hypomagnesemia can cause hypocalcemia due to impaired secretion of parathyroid hormone, her hypermagnesemia is not contributing. Hyperphosphatemia may cause hypocalcemia because of local precipitation of calcium-phosphate salts. Her hypophosphatemia is not the cause of the hypocalcemia. Thiazide diuretics are associated with hypercalcemia, not hypocalcemia. Primary hyperparathyroidism causes hypercalcemia, not hypocalcemia.

288. Answer: C

The correct answer is discontinue his oral agents for glycemic control and switch him to insulin. This question requires you to know that triglyceride levels are very dependent upon glycemic control. This patient has gained a significant amount of weight and his insulin resistance has worsened to the point that he is not controlled on the combination of a thiazolidinedione, metformin, and a rapid-acting secretagogue, despite taking the maximum allowable doses. At this point, he must be switched to insulin. His triglyceride level was much better 6 months ago when his glycemic control was better. It is safe to assume that the increase in triglyceride levels is due to his worsening control. This scenario is commonly seen with diabetic patients. Before specifically targeting his triglyceride levels, his glycemic control must first be improved.

Adding a fibrate to a statin is controversial. Though some physicians do it, the combination is not approved by the FDA at the time of this writing. In fact, a statin drug was dropped because of adverse events in patients prescribed the combination. A fibrate could certainly be used once the statin was discontinued, but a fibrate is not as good an agent at lowering LDL cholesterol. His LDL was 170 mg/dL in the past. It is unlikely that his LDL will remain controlled once he has been switched from a statin to a fibrate. An α-glucosidase inhibitor is expected to lower HbA1c by about 0.5 percentage points. This will not provide enough control for his hyperglycemia. Moreover, there are no quadruple combinations approved by the FDA. In fact, there are no triple-combinations currently approved. Besides, there is some evidence that an α-glucosidase inhibitor will inhibit absorption of some other oral agents and this area requires more investigation. Adding a second statin will not help the situation. If anything, this will increase his risk of an adverse event.

289. Answer: A

The correct answer is begin dexamethasone 1 mg IV every 8 hours and order an ACTH stimulation test. There is a strong suspicion that this patient has adrenal insufficiency and is having an adrenal crisis. She is hypovolemic with a hyperkalemic metabolic acidosis. The hypotension responded well to saline fluids. The thin body habitus and loss of axillary and pubic hair imply a chronic adrenal insufficiency. The flight delay may have caused stress for some reason that she was not able to cope with because of the adrenal insufficiency. This may have been what tipped her over the edge. Whether she really has an adrenal crisis or not is not the issue. It is more important to begin treatment than it is to prove your suspicion. The treatment is to give her intravenous glucocorticoids as soon as possible. But which glucocorticoid should you give? Remember, you do not yet have proof of the adrenal insufficiency. You can start treatment based on a suspicion, but you must also pursue a diagnosis. The diagnostic workup begins with an ACTH stimulation test. To do this, order a baseline serum cortisol level, administer 1 ampule of ACTH, and repeat the cortisol level 30 minutes later. The important thing to remember is that the assay for cortisol will cross-react with most other glucocorticoids and also pick up prednisone, methylprednisolone, and especially hydrocortisone since it is cortisol under a different name. If any of these are administered, how will you know what her endogenous production of cortisol really is? The solution is to administer a glucocorticoid that does not interfere with the cortisol assay, such as dexamethasone. She needs a glucocorticoid to save her life; begin dexamethasone immediately. If her adrenal function proves to be okay, you can easily stop the steroid. To check her adrenal function, check for her response to ACTH. If the cortisol level is greater than 20 µg/dL, her adrenal reserve is intact and you can stop the dexamethasone. If the ACTH stimulation test shows adrenal insufficiency, stop the dexamethasone and switch her to hydrocortisone. This is the actual cortisol molecule and it has an advantage over the other glucocorticoids. Hydrocortisone (cortisol) is primarily a glucocorticoid, but it also has some mineralocorticoid activity that will help with her electrolytes.

The other answers are incorrect because a glucocorticoid other than dexamethasone should not be used for the above reasons. Hypothyroidism is unlikely, so starting thyroxine is not indicated. Once her adrenal crisis has resolved, you can re-evaluate her.

290. Answer: C

The correct answer is fluid restriction to 800 cc/hour. As SIADH is due to increased effect of ANTI-diuretic hormone, treatment must compensate for the excess fluid retention by delivering LESS fluid. No other treatment works quickly. The ultimate goal is to eradicate or shrink the tumor so it produces less ADH-like material. Definitive treatment of the underlying cause of excess ADH is slow compared to the rapid correction achieved by water restriction. One can create renal loss of fluid by inducing nephrogenic diabetes insipidus with demeclocycline (900-1200 mg/d). This creates a compensatory pathology, when the underlying cause of inappropriate renal fluid retention cannot be corrected. (Like pouring cold water on someone caught in the desert rather than taking them out of the heat.) Desmopressin is an antidiuretic hormone and the patient already has too much of this; it's a good "bait" answer because it sounds similar to the correct answer and is in the pituitary chapter. Avoid hypertonic saline except in life-threatening hyponatremia…it has many hazards and should be used in the ICU only.

291. Answer: B

The correct answer is dopamine agonist. Whenever a woman has not had menses, exclude pregnancy with serum beta-HCG. DO NOT forget this test in any patient with abdominal pain…ruptured ectopic pregnancy is a favorite board question as is ruptured spleen, but I digress. Severe hypothyroidism (i.e., with TSH over 50) can cause pituitary enlargement and hyperprolactinemia that resolve with thyroxine administration. If the TSH is markedly elevated, there is no need for a T4 or the other serum tests. Because the prolactin level is below 100- 200, your suspicion for co-secretory or an extremely large pituitary adenoma interrupting the dopamine inhibitory paths in the pituitary stalk should be high and therefore you should obtain the additional tests. Prolactinomas can co-secrete human growth hormone (hGH). The treatment of acromegaly with prolactinoma is surgical so it must be excluded. Hopefully, this degree of sophistication will not be expected for the boards…remember it in practice, however. MRI gives the best sella definition, especially as she may have a very small prolactinoma. Excluding Cushing's disease is important because it causes menstrual disruption and can be the first recognized symptom. If she has a large pituitary tumor, the T4 would be low due to inadequate TSH-secretory reserve. Do NOT forget medication history in all clinical case questions. The physiology that the hyperprolactinemic state disrupts is ovarian cycling: therefore, infertility and low estrogen state with potential for endometrial hyperplasia (as the progesterone surge and its consequent endometrial deciduation is suppressed), osteopenia, and loss of estrogen's cardio protection. If the tumor enlarges sufficiently it can cause visual field loss. This is one time when anatomy becomes as important as FUNCTION in endocrine evaluation.

292. Answer: C

The correct "incorrect" answer is Headache. Pituitary tumors are secretory and hyperplasia of all the cell types has been reported: TSH, ACTH, hGH, gonadotrophins, and prolactin. Through mass effect a nonsecretory or secretory adenoma can cause deficiency in the production of the other hormones, especially TSH and ACTH. Headache is almost never caused by or when present relieved by treatment for a pituitary adenoma.

293. Answer: E

The correct answer is Thyroid scan and uptake. You need to know thyroid FUNCTION, not its anatomy. The absence of symptoms due to mass effect from the thyroid: e.g., no recurrent laryngeal nerve impingement (i.e., no voice change, weakness or "gravelly" sound), no dysphagia or dyspnea exclude the need for anatomic studies: CT, ultrasound, and scan. Obtaining a thyroid scan and uptake (which reveal the gland's FUNCTIONAL ability to concentration I-131), you find diminished uptake except in the left lower pole of the thyroid where there is a "hot" nodule.

294. Answer: A

The correct answer is atorvastatin. The point here is that he needs LDL treated, and if possible, HDL raised. He is already exercising, which is an excellent means to raise HDL. Niacin would be a good choice as well; the boards should not make you choose between atorvastatin and niacin to lower LDL and raise HDL as there is no clear consensus as to which is preferable.

In caring for hyperlipidemia differentiating between isolated elevation of LDL, versus isolated triglycerides or a mixture of elevated triglycerides and LDL is critical. Each circumstance has different treatment strategies. See the Core Curriculum for treatment guidelines.

295. Answer: C

The correct answer is Cortrosyn stimulation. This is a classic presentation for Addison's disease, the disease that almost kept John F. Kennedy out of the White House. She has fatigue, asthenia and listlessness, and recurrent flu-like illnesses. Further history may be that of a family history of autoimmune endocrine disorders (Type 1 diabetes, Hashimoto's disease, Graves' disease) or of tuberculosis she acquired overseas if it had been left untreated…but that is too convoluted for the boards. The Cortrosyn stimulation is the diagnostic test and should be done next. Screening for other autoimmune endocrine disorders is reasonable, but not a priority. This is not the history of bulimia so a dental screening for enamel etching due to vomiting is not necessary. Treatment should be a corticosteroid and mineralocorticoid, as the aldosterone-producing cells are often involved to some extent.

296. Answer: D

The correct answer is adrenal cancer. This question asks you to know two things: late onset and rapid progression of androgenization means cancer. The ovary is the major source of measured testosterone in the woman; the adrenal is the major producer of DHEA, so extraordinarily high DHEA-S means adrenal cancer. To evaluate hirsutism requires DHEA-S and testosterone. If the hirsutism is milder and insidious with symptoms beginning in puberty or the early twenties, it is more likely due to PCOS, LH: FSH ratio over 2.5 along with high normal or above normal testosterone occurs. There is controversy about establishing the diagnosis, so ovarian ultrasound (not a FUNCTIONAL test) is not required. This question asks you to know two things about appropriate treatment for adrenal carcinoma: prompt excision and poor prognosis.

297. Answer: B

The correct answer is Klinefelter's syndrome. This exam points toward eunuchoid development with span greater than height, which is compatible with late epiphyseal closure due to underproduction of testosterone, and the gynecomastia also points toward relative insufficient testosterone production. The key is the small (usually described as firm) testes and gynecomastia, which point to Klinefelter's syndrome. Kallmann's syndrome is not correct because congenital hypogonadotropic hypogonadism has low amounts of both estrogens and testosterone so gynecomastia does not develop.

298. Answer: E

The correct answer is to increase the supper Humalog and decrease the bedtime NPH. You are asked to recognize that erratic fasting glucoses may represent unrecognized nocturnal hypoglycemia, and cut her bedtime NPH.

299. Answer: B

The correct answer is diet, daily walks, and ACE inhibitor. Beyond diet and exercise, ACE inhibitors are warranted to control hypertension to 120's over 80's and give renal protection. You would wait on treating the diabetes until you had seen how diet and exercise worked.

300. Answer: A

The correct answer is metformin. For a consistently elevated fasting glucose with diet modification, metformin is indicated to diminish hepatic gluconeogenesis. It is the first-step treatment for Type 2 diabetes.

301. Answer: C

The correct answer is symptoms of hypoglycemia, low serum glucose, and symptom relief with glucose. This question asks you to understand causes of hypoglycemia, and differentiate between fasting (insulinoma) and post-prandial (dumping syndrome and "reactive") hypoglycemia. Once you discriminate between hypoglycemia, which occurs in the fasting state that is due to insulin excess—endogenous or exogenous and that which occurs after eating, the correct diagnosis is post-gastrectomy syndrome. Also, it is necessary to remember that Whipple's triad of hypoglycemic symptoms occurs during periods of low serum glucose and is relieved by a source of sugar.

302. Answer: E

The correct answer is Paget's disease. It causes an asymptomatic elevation of alkaline phosphatase most commonly. As the patients can be asymptomatic or have aching that is similar in quality to the pain of DJD, indications for intervention are important to know: encroachment on neuro foramen, CHF from increased blood flow, threat to weight-bearing bones, and pain are reasons for treatment.

303. Answer: B

The correct answer is that the growth hormone concentration should NOT be suppressed in his condition, which is growth hormone excess. He presents with the clinical syndrome of acromegaly with bony and soft tissue overgrowth, enlargement of the jaw and tongue, wide spacing of the teeth, and coarsened facial features. Hypertension may result because of expansion of the plasma volume and total body sodium. A moist, oily doughy handshake is characteristic.

Laboratory findings include abnormal glucose tolerance and mild hyperprolactinemia. The reason for growth hormone excess in almost all patients with acromegaly is a pituitary adenoma. Useful screening tests include measurements of glucose-suppressed growth hormone concentrations (which normally is suppressed to below 1 microgram/L) and IGF binding protein 3. IGF-I concentrations are elevated secondary to the high levels of growth hormone. Once you have confirmed acromegaly or have a good suspicion, you should proceed to MRI to find the pituitary adenoma.

304. Answer: D

The correct answer is that Graves's disease is UNLIKELY! You were thinking all along that it was Graves, right? Well, that stupid radioactive iodine uptake test threw that answer out—with Graves it is never LOW. The thyrotoxic phase of subacute and silent thyroiditis is associated with an inflammatory breakdown and release of stored thyroid hormone, which will feed back onto the hypothalamus and anterior pituitary to inhibit TSH secretion. This will produce a low RAIU for a while. Struma ovarii, remember, consists of ectopic hyperfunctioning autonomous thyroid tissue—like in a teratoma, which also will result in a low RAIU in the thyroid (the pelvis is scanned though and would show an INCREASED uptake here). Iodine-induced thyrotoxicosis will generally occur in the face of a preexisting dysfunctional thyroid. We see this mainly in someone who is coming from a country with low iodine intake and then they come to the great USA with our HIGH iodine intakes.

305. Answer: C

The correct answer is to do nothing at this point. This guy has Familial Hypocalciuric Hypercalcemia (FHH), also known as benign familial hypercalcemia. This consists of an elevated serum calcium, normal or low serum phosphorus, a normal or high serum PTH, a slightly elevated magnesium, and a low urinary calcium excretion. This is inherited as an autosomal dominant disorder of chromosomes 3 or 19. No therapy is required—remember, a favorite of the ABIM.

Surgery will not correct the hypercalcemia. The other thing to be careful about is that these patients can be misdiagnosed as hyperparathyroidism if the urinary calcium is not measured. Untreated these patients generally remain asymptomatic without evidence of renal calculi, HTN, or other problems with hypercalcemia.

---

306. Answer: B

The correct answer is that she has tertiary hyperparathyroidism. This is seen commonly in renal patients where the parathyroid glands become autonomous. The hypercalcemia develops gradually over time and is rarely life threatening. It is associated with osteitis fibrosa. It can be treated with aluminum "binders." Finally, parathyroid hormone half-life is actually INCREASED in renal insufficiency.

---

307. Answer: A

The correct answer is radioactive iodine uptake. This post partum female has symptoms and lab work suggesting hyperthyroidism. The most common cause in this setting would be post partum thyroiditis. The most definitive test to rule out the alternative diagnosis of Grave's disease would be a 24 hour radioactive iodine uptake. Patients with Grave's disease have a high 24 hour radioiodine uptake, whereas patients with acute or subacute thyroiditis have a very low radioiodine uptake.

---

308. Answer: D

The correct answer is interaction between levothyroxine sodium and $FeSO_4$. This patient has a history of hypothyroidism treated with levothyroxine. She develops iron-deficiency anemia and is started on iron. She then develops symptoms and signs of hypothyroidism: dry skin, elevated cholesterol, constipation, and muscle pain. The reason for her hypothyroidism is poor absorption of the levothyroxine she is taking because of an interaction between the oral iron she is taking and the levothyroxine.

---

309. Answer: E

The correct answer is coumarin administration. Increased PT with a normal PTT and platelets usually indicates coumarin administration. Factor VII deficiency could do this also.

---

310. Answer: B

The correct answer is CBC with platelet count, PT, PTT, and bleeding time. Note that coagulation factor deficiencies are more likely to present with complications such as hemarthrosis. Platelet disorders usually present with mucosal bleeding and a history of bleeding with light trauma. Doing more than the initial workup outlined is "overkill." Knowing what the PTT, PT, and platelet counts are will help guide the direction in which you need to proceed.

---

311. Answer: C

The correct answer is chronic myelogenous leukemia (CML). I know this is a "simple" knowledge question, but believe it or not, they will ask you this one somewhere on the test. They are likely to give you a scenario of someone you diagnose this in and then ask you to name the chromosomal abnormality associated with this disease. So, bottom line—KNOW IT!!!!!!

312. Answer: A

The correct answer is hereditary spherocytosis. The clues here are the splenomegaly at age 20 (pretty much rules out Sickle cell disease—remember they auto-splenectomize) and the elevated MCHC, increased osmotic fragility, and the decreased red cell survival. The history of gallstones in relatives at early ages is also common in this disease. It is quite common and occurs in 1/5000 in northern Europeans.

313. Answer: D

The correct answer is a cutaneous vasculitis may also appear in this condition. The patient has hairy cell leukemia. It frequently can be difficult to discern from polyarteritis. Neutropenia is quite common, as well as pancytopenia. The disease is associated with both defects in humoral and cellular immunity and will respond to alpha-interferon. Splenectomy will not be curative, as it will not affect the marrow. The cytoplasmic projections are classic for this disease process.

314. Answer: B

The correct answer is hepatitis B virus is serving as a helper for a viral superinfection. In this case, it is likely that he has developed a superinfection with hepatitis D. Hepatitis D requires the hepatitis B genome to replicate. Hepatitis C and A cannot facilitate hepatitis D infection. Interferon alpha will not be curative for the superinfection, but may help alleviate some of the symptoms.

315. Answer: B

The correct answer is protein C deficiency. Coumarin-induced skin necrosis has been well described in patients with protein C deficiency. The skin lesions most commonly occur on the breasts, buttocks, and legs. The penis is also a described site. The theory is that an imbalance in homeostasis occurs, favoring thrombosis during the early phases of coumarin administration. We know that protein C has a short half life of about 14 hours compared to some of the vitamin-K dependent factors such as factor X—and a rapid drop in the protein C concentration could produce this scenario.

316. Answer: C

The correct answer is α-thalassemia trait. This occurs when people have deletion of 2 of the 4 alpha-chain genes. These individuals tend to have a microcytic and slightly hypochromic red cell, but without significant anemia or hemolysis. Hemoglobin electrophoresis can be normal or may show a decreased amount of hemoglobin A2. All of the other abnormalities listed would have microcytosis, but the hemoglobin electrophoresis would be abnormal.

317. Answer: E

The correct answer is hydration and analgesia. She is having a sickle cell pain crisis that can be frequently precipitated by an upper respiratory infection or dehydration. It can be very difficult to distinguish from a crisis and an acute abdomen, so vigilance must be observed. Hydration is the key initially!! Hydroxyurea may reduce the incidence of sickle crises by increasing synthesis of fetal hemoglobin, but has no role in an acute crisis.

Antibiotics would only be administered if an infection was documented. Chest syndrome is something to be very concerned about in this patient and would require aggressive monitoring of her condition.

318. Answer: A

The correct answer is to stop PTU and schedule a follow-up appointment. She most likely has severe neutropenia as an idiosyncratic reaction to PTU. She is at risk for overwhelming, life-threatening infection, but at the moment without signs of fever or other signs of infection, she can be followed as an outpatient. Steroids are not useful in this setting. You would never continue the offending drug. Almost always, severe drug-induced neutropenia reverses fairly quickly and therefore consideration for bone marrow transplant is not indicated at this point.

319. Answer: D

The correct answer is plasmapheresis. This woman has thrombocytopenic purpura (TTP). You can put this together very easily: Hemolytic anemia with fragmented red cells, thrombocytopenia, fever, mental status changes, and renal dysfunction WITHOUT evidence of disseminated intravascular coagulation (DIC) is classic for TTP. Plasmapheresis or exchange transfusion is the preferred treatment.

320. Answer: B

The correct "incorrect" answer is intravascular hemolysis has likely occurred. This presentation is consistent with a delayed transfusion reaction. Immediate transfusion reactions that would manifest as intravascular hemolysis are most commonly due to ABO incompatibility. Usually these are due to clerical error. Fever, malaise, and a drop in hematocrit 1 week after red cell transfusion are typical of delayed transfusion reactions, which are usually mediated by antibodies to Rh unless the patient is Rh-negative, then it is mediated by antibodies to anti-Duffy, Anti-Kell, or Anti-Kidd. These antibodies coat the donor red cells, which results in a positive direct Coombs' test. Less commonly, the donor's plasma could contain antibodies that could react with the recipient's cells. (WHEW! Doesn't this stuff just drive you crazy!)

321. Answer: C

The correct answer is she has developed alloantibodies in her serum. Patients who receive a large number of transfusions frequently will develop a large panel of alloantibodies. This makes it difficult to type and match appropriate blood for these patients. The presence of these antibodies may or may not produce hemolysis if blood containing a potential target antigen is transfused; however, blood banks will not allow transfusion of these products unless it is an emergency situation.

322. Answer: A

The correct answer is severe hypokalemia. This may occur early in the course of therapy. This represents a return of potassium to intracellular sites. Reticulocytosis is usually brisk and is a hallmark of correct diagnosis and treatment of this disease.

323. Answer: D

The correct answer is folate in large doses can correct the megaloblastic anemia, but it does not correct the neurologic abnormalities. Antiparietal-cell antibodies are common and seen in 90% of those with pernicious anemia. Gastrin levels are usually elevated in those with pernicious anemia.

324. Answer: E

The correct answer is impaired transfer of reticuloendothelial storage iron to marrow erythroid precursors. The anemia of chronic disease is usually a normochromic, normocytic anemia. Bone marrow examination will show normal red cell maturation. Hemolysis does not usually occur. Hemoglobin synthesis is usually normal also. Patients usually have a low serum iron and a low total transferrin level. Storage iron is usually quite abundant. However, there is a decreased amount of iron in erythroblasts—this indicates a defect in the transfer of reticuloendothelial iron to immature red blood cells.

325. Answer: C

The correct answer is hemolysis is commonly induced by infection. Viruses or bacterial infection are most common and they induce an environmental oxidant stress. Drugs such as dapsone, sulfonamides, antimalarial agents, and vitamin K can also trigger hemolysis. The gene for G6PD is on the X-chromosome; therefore, it is a sex-linked trait. Men are more commonly involved than women. The Mediterranean variant is more severe than the A-type, which is found in the majority of African-Americans. The Heinz bodies can only been seen with special supravital stains. G6PD levels decrease as the red cell ages. So, during an acute episode of hemolysis, it is a bad time to check for the deficiency as a false-negative test will be seen as the newer cells being made during hemolysis will have higher levels of G6PD than older cells.

326. Answer: B

The correct answer is normochromic, normocytic red blood cells. You would expect a very low reticulocyte count, not an elevated one. The bone marrow examination in pure red cell aplasia contrasts with aplastic anemia in that you expect to find a normocellular or hypercellular marrow in patients with pure red cell aplasia. Ferrokinetic studies would show a reduced iron turnover. Erythropoietin levels would be elevated in red cell aplasia.

327. Answer: E

The correct answer is to check Factor VII levels. The finding of a prolonged PT and a normal PTT suggests a defect in the extrinsic coagulation cascade. Factor VII deficiency is RARE and is autosomal recessive: however, looking at the choices this is the best test to order. Remember on the Boards—go with what is the best possible answer! Factor VIII deficiency as well as the presence of coagulation factor inhibitors (Factor VIII inhibitor is the most common) would prolong the PTT. An α_2–antiplasmin deficiency results in a bleeding disorder with accelerated clot lysis; the PT and PTT are normal in these patients.

328. Answer: D

The correct answer is that hemolytic uremic syndrome would be least likely to produce a thrombocytosis. Remember that it is a disease most common in children and results in a condition similar to thrombotic thrombocytopenic purpura! Thrombocytopenia is very common in hemolytic uremic syndrome. All of the other conditions/diseases listed would be more likely to produce a thrombocytosis.

329. Answer: C

The correct answer is aspirin. She has von Willebrand's disease and using aspirin would further aggravate her ability to aggregate platelet response. The other drugs listed are not contraindicated in von Willebrand's. Even if you didn't have a clue what the heck was going on in this question—aspirin makes the most sense—of the choices listed aspirin has a known effect on platelets; therefore if you are "in the dark" on a question pick something that seems "obvious" and go for it—or go for the most obscure thing if you really don't have a clue—maybe they are trying to let you "learn" on the examination by asking you about some zebra (much less likely than the "obvious" choice though!).

330. Answer: A

The correct answer is Factor XII deficiency. Platelet deficiency will result in normal PT and PTT except bleeding time will be abnormal. von Willebrand's will result in normal PT and PTT, but an abnormally prolonged bleeding time with normal platelet aggregation. Factor VII deficiency will result in abnormal prolongation of the PT but a normal PTT. Glanzmann thrombasthenia will result in a normal PT and PTT but an abnormal bleeding time, as well as abnormal platelet aggregation.

331. Answer: D

The correct answer is patients lack glycoprotein 1b. Patients have severely decreased platelet adhesion because of the lack of glycoprotein 1b. The platelets cannot bind to von Willebrand Factor. They usually have a modestly low platelet count also. It is an autosomal recessive disease.

332. Answer: B

The correct answer is it is due to a deficiency of glycoprotein IIb-IIIa complex. This is an autosomal recessive disorder. The lack of this glycoprotein complex does NOT permit fibrinogen to cross-connect, resulting in severe bleeding. Platelet counts are usually normal in this disease.

333. Answer: E

The correct answer is iron deficiency anemia. She has the classic symptoms and findings. Her history of menorrhagia is common and frequently results in iron deficiency anemia in younger women. The other diagnoses at her age are very unlikely. Remember, common things are common and rare things are rare.

334. Answer: C

The correct answer is myelodysplastic syndrome is UNLIKELY. Myelodysplastic syndrome is usually seen in elderly patients (she is quite young) and is characterized by HIGH MCVs and hypercellular bone marrows. Iron deficiency anemia will give you a low MCV with anemia as she has. In the anemia of chronic disease you usually have a normal MCV but it can be low on occasion. The thalassemias (alpha and beta) will produce a microcytic anemia as she has. Sideroblastic anemia is rare but would have these findings.

335. Answer: E

The correct answer is alcoholism is most likely the cause of his anemia. By definition he has a macrocytic anemia. Luckily, only a few things will do this: alcoholism (due to interference with folic acid metabolism), B_{12} deficiency, myelodysplastic syndrome, etc. Vitamin B_{12} deficiency is relatively rare and with his current diet is unlikely to develop. Myelodysplastic syndrome occurs in his age group, but is less common and we see evidence of liver disease with the presence of target cells, as well as the mildly elevated transaminases. Iron deficiency anemia would not give this picture.

336. Answer: C

The correct answer is hairy cell leukemia. Note that hairy cell leukemia is a neoplasm of mature B-lymphocytes typically presenting with pancytopenia, splenomegaly, and a dry bone marrow aspirate. Patients with hairy cell are prone to infections with unusual organisms like atypical mycobacteria. Bone marrow findings can include "fried egg" appearance in that cells appear to be separated from each other due to the "projections and fixation artifacts" generated by the hairy cells. It is easily treated and responds well to chemotherapy. Pancytopenia with a dry tap go against CLL and myeloma. Normal RBC morphology goes against myelofibrosis. The WBC and differential go against CML.

337. Answer: A

The correct answer is hepatic venography. He most likely has polycythemia rubra vera with the presence of primary erythrocytosis with organomegaly. A complication of this disorder is hypercoagulability, with hepatic vein thrombosis being a particular problem seen. Hepatic vein thrombosis would lead to Budd-Chiari syndrome where you would have a grossly enlarged liver with severe ascites. The best way to diagnosis this is by hepatic venography or liver biopsy where you would look for sinusoidal dilatation.

338. Answer: D

The correct answer is Factor XIII deficiency. This disorder may be inherited or acquired and frequently causes severe bleeding problems. In this disorder, the bleeding time, PT, and PTT are all normal!! The screening test for factor XIII deficiency is checking a "clot solubility in urea assay". People with Factor XII and prekallikrein deficiency also have prolongation of PTT but do not have problems with surgery. Normal bleeding time excludes thrombasthenia, an inherited disorder of platelet aggregation. Protein S is a vitamin K-dependent plasma protein and a cofactor for expression of the anticoagulant activity of activated protein C.

339. Answer: B

The correct answer is that normal levels of protein C rules out the disease—this is INCORRECT!!!!!!!!!!! Protein C is an anticoagulant that inactivates clotting factors V and VII. When deficient it can lead to thrombosis commonly of the lower extremity deep veins as well as the iliofemoral or mesenteric veins. The majority are spontaneous while the rest occur in association with a stress such as surgery or pregnancy. It is inherited as an autosomal dominant disease. Two forms of the disease exist: 1) normal levels of protein C but they are a biologically dysfunctional protein, and 2) deficient levels. Therefore, just measuring the level of protein C will not "rule out" the disease. You must also measure "tests of function." Besides the inherited form, acquired protein C deficiency can occur. This can happen with DIC, severe liver disease, nephrotic syndrome, etc.

340. Answer: E

The correct answer is protamine sulfate. Protamine sulfate is INAPPROPRIATE. She has warfarin-induced skin necrosis due to protein C deficiency. She probably has acquired the disease from her liver dysfunction. The cutaneous vessels thrombose when warfarin was added without heparin. Since protein C has a short half-life, warfarin inactivates this protein before any of the other clotting factors. This can lead to a temporary procoagulant state that is exacerbated in a patient who is already deficient in protein C. If immediate intervention is not begun, the lesion will spread and she will develop skin necrosis. Treatment is to stop warfarin and start heparin. You also should administer vitamin K to counteract any further effect warfarin may be having. If all this fails, then giving protein C concentrate or protein C-containing products such as fresh frozen plasma should be given. Protamine counteracts heparin and is contraindicated.

341. Answer: D

The correct answer is B_{12} deficiency. This patient has Zollinger-Ellison syndrome, which is managed through the use of high dose proton pump inhibitors. High doses of proton pump inhibitors can decrease absorption of vitamin B_{12}. Oral B_{12} absorption is reduced by 90% in volunteers taking 40 mg of Omeprazole.

342. Answer: A

The correct answer is to remove the central venous catheter and start empiric broad-spectrum antibiotics as well as amphotericin B. In this severely neutropenic woman, as well as her overwhelmingly immunocompromised state from her recent transplant and medications, all bacterial etiologies as well as severe fungemias must be considered particularly with *Candida* species. Therefore it is reasonable to start broad-spectrum antibiotics as well as amphotericin B initially. The line must be removed at any sign of infection particularly if fungal infection is suspected as in this woman.

343. Answer: B

The correct answer is that a change in the color of the lesion warrants further workup for potential malignancy. One of the characteristics that distinguishes a superficial spreading malignant melanoma from a normal mole is a change in the color of the lesion. Another warning sign is if the border becomes irregular. Usually the first change noted is a "darkening" in color or a change in the borders of the lesion. Excisional biopsy should be done promptly because early diagnosis and excision reduce mortality.

344. Answer: D

The correct answer is bronchoscopy, esophagoscopy, and laryngoscopy. A firm neck mass in a smoker and heavy drinker always is suspicious for squamous cell carcinoma of the head and neck. The finding of squamous cell carcinoma on the biopsy warrants an aggressive search for a primary lesion in the head and neck region and therefore the multiple endoscopies are indicated. CT of the neck would help with determining the extent of the disease but is unlikely to reveal the primary. Once a primary is determined and the extent of the disease then the decision on therapy can be made. Standard therapy for primary head and neck squamous cell carcinoma with lymph node metastasis is radiation therapy, surgery, or both. Adjuvant chemotherapy is being investigated to reduce tumor load before surgery or radiation.

345. Answer: A

The correct answer is that cystic fibrosis is NOT associated with development of malignancy. Fanconi's anemia is associated with cytogenetic abnormalities and has an increased risk of cancer. Approximately 10% of patients with neurofibromatosis develop sarcomatous changes. Ataxia-telangiectasia is associated with lymphoma. Familial polyposis coli predisposes to colon cancer in all patients with this disorder.

346. Answer: C

The correct answer is anthracycline agents suppress bone marrow stem cells to a greater degree than they do more "committed" hematopoietic cells is a false statement. The anthracycline agents generally suppress the more "committed" cells than the stem cell lines. The other statements are correct. Cisplatin causes large renal loses of potassium and magnesium that in turn leads to hypocalcemia. Vincristine is a relatively mild myelosuppressive agent and can be used in periods of low white blood cell counts.

347. Answer: E

The correct answer is to administer leuprolide and flutamide—anti-androgen therapy. Anti-androgen therapy is at least as effective as orchiectomy and will spare him surgery as well as the complications of surgery. Knowing that he had poorly differentiated disease at initial diagnosis and now the findings of bone lesions in his ribs and pelvis, biopsy is not necessary. Prostate cancer is not very responsive to chemotherapy such as cisplatin.

348. Answer: B

The correct answer is bone scan; as it would not be helpful for this disease—Multiple Myeloma. Myeloma causes osteolytic lesions not osteoblastic lesions—remember a bone scan can only pick up osteoblastic lesions. The skeletal survey would be very helpful in determining extent of disease as would the β_2-microglobulin. Renal involvement is quite common with multiple myeloma and determination of 24-hour urine protein excretion can be helpful in determining prognosis. Serum protein electrophoresis is also helpful in diagnosis.

349. Answer: B

The correct answer is ovarian cancer of germ cell lineage. Most ovarian cancers are of epithelial cell lineage however she had evidence of hormonal abnormalities with the hirsutism, deepening voice, and clitorimegaly. All of these findings are consistent with virilization and androgen production. These ovarian germ cell tumors can be treated similarly to testicular carcinoma in men and respond to therapy with cisplatin and etoposide.

350. Answer: E

The correct answer is Mantle Cell lymphoma. For the Boards, I would know this lymphoma. Frankly though I never heard of it (but then I did residency pre-1990). It is now WELL-DESCRIBED in the literature and we used to call it intermediate lymphoma. The key with this lymphoma is the immunophenotypical characteristics: The cells express B-cell antigens such as CD19 and CD20 as well as the nominal T-Cell antigen CD5. This B-cell lymphoma is one of the only B-cell lymphomas to express this antigen! Chronic lymphocytic leukemia will do it too! (sounds like board material to me). Additionally the t(11;14) translocation is nearly always associated with mantle cell lymphoma! (Ditto on Board Relevance!) What does the t(11;14) translocation do you may ask? It brings cyclin D_1 under the influence of immunoglobulin heavy chain promoters and leads to cyclin D_1 over expression. (Now, aren't you sorry you asked?? YES!! What ever that means). But remember for the Boards: CD19, CD20 and CD5 positivity and t(11;14) translocation mean Mantle Cell Lymphoma!!

351. Answer: A

The correct answer is he has entered an accelerated or blastic phase. The Philadelphia chromosome is the diagnostic "hallmark" of chronic myeloid leukemia. Remember that it involves the translocation between chromosome 22 and chromosome 9. Patients with CML usually have a chronic benign phase for 3-4 years. The most commonly observed cytogenetic event to signify an accelerated or blast phase is duplication of the Philadelphia chromosome!

352. Answer: C

The correct answer is to substitute controlled-release morphine 60 to 120 mg twice a day in place of her oxycodone. A majority of patients with advanced cancer experience pain that may be caused by tumor invasion, surgical procedures or due to radiation/chemotherapy agents. Most can experience pain control with the proper agents. In this woman with moderately severe pain, it is reasonable to place her on a more potent drug at a higher dose such as controlled-release morphine.

353. Answer: D

The correct answer is early onset coronary artery disease. Within months of mantle irradiation about 15% develop LOWER extremity paresthesia upon flexion of the neck, also known as Lhermitte's sign. Radiation pneumonitis is also a concern in a small percentage of patients (<5%). Other complications of mantle radiation include pericardial effusion, myocardial injury and an increased risk of coronary artery disease. Hypothyroidism occurs in over 80% of patients! Breast cancer and lung cancer are increased in incidence as well as stomach, skin and soft tissue sarcomas. Acute leukemias are rare in patients not treated with chemotherapy agents.

354. Answer: A

The correct answer is biopsy. Cervical cancer mortality is so preventable because it is easily revealed by the Pap smear. But it's only a screening test. If the Pap returns with low-grade squamous intraepithelial lesion (or high-grade) then a punch biopsy is required for diagnosis of CIN or invasive carcinoma. If the biopsy then shows CIN I (slight dysplasia) this may resolve, and does not require treatment. Followup with a repeat Pap smear in 4-6 months. CIN II and III (moderate and severe dysplasia) are treated with ablative therapy, either cryotherapy or laser. If the punch biopsy returns showing invasive carcinoma, staging is done, and the patient is treated with hysterectomy or radiation, or both. If the biopsy did not make the stage of the pre malignancy clear, then conization is indicated.

355. Answer: B

The correct answer is serous or mucinous epithelial cancer. The diagnosis, considering the patient's age, her BRCA1 associated risk, and elevated CA-125 is almost certainly ovarian cancer. Half of all ovarian cancer patients are over age 65, and there is a 40% lifetime risk of ovarian cancer associated with the presence of BRCA1 (compared to 1.5% risk in the female population.) The BRCA1 gene, found in 5% of women, is also associated with a 50 to 80% lifetime risk of developing breast cancer. The CA-125 is commonly increased in ovarian cancer, and should be obtained in any patient suspected of having this disease. Serous and mucinous epithelial carcinomas are by far the most common ovarian cancers. (85% of ovarian cancer is epithelial cell, half of these serous, and 1/4 mucinous.) Germ cell cancers, including choriocarcinoma, usually occur in younger patients, and can elevate both alpha fetoprotein and HCG. These two levels are not increased in epithelial carcinoma. Clear cell carcinoma, another epithelial cell type, is uncommon.

356. Answer: B

The correct answer is radiotherapy & chemotherapy & tamoxifen. Although this is a small tumor -- less than a centimeter -- the presence of a positive axillary node means that she should receive adjuvant therapy as if it were large. Because the tumor was found to be HR+, both chemotherapy and tamoxifen are recommended. All lumpectomies include node dissection and should be followed with radiotherapy in order to be "the equivalent" of a mastectomy. Chemotherapy and Tamoxifen should be used without radiation only if a mastectomy is done -- when premenopausal and HR+, or postmenopausal with more than one positive node and HR+. Tamoxifen as a sole agent can be used only if the patient is postmenopausal, a modified radical mastectomy is done, no positive nodes are found, and the tumor is HR+.

357. Answer: B

The correct answer is seminoma. Seminomas comprise 60% of germ cell tumors, and non seminomas the remaining 40%. Germ cell tumors comprise 95% of all testicular tumors. Sertoli cell cancer is uncommon. Torsion is an acute process accompanied by intense pain and tenderness. Hydroceles are cystic, not solid or firm.

358. Answer: A

The correct answer is acute myelogenous leukemia (AML). All of the other malignancies will usually result in splenomegaly. This can be helpful when trying to differentiate AML from the other entities.

359. Answer: B

The correct answer is acute myelogenous leukemia (AML). AML is unusual in that lymphadenopathy is NOT common. Splenomegaly also is NOT common in AML.

360. Answer: B

The correct answer is acute myelogenous leukemia. She has gingival hyperplasia!! And she doesn't have an enlarged spleen. The gingival hyperplasia is seen in nearly ½ of patients with monocytic AML (M5). The others are unlikely to do this. Jean-Luke Picard syndrome does not cause acute leukemia..in fact I don't think it does anything cause I just made it up while watching some television show.

361. Answer: D

The correct answer is neurotoxicity. These patients can develop a peripheral neuropathy.

362. Answer: C

The correct answer is on immunophenotyping, CD11c marker is likely to be present. Bone marrow aspirate in Hairy cell leukemia is usually DRY despite the fact that you have a HYPERCELLULAR bone marrow on biopsy. This is due to increased reticulin. 2-CdA will induce a complete remission in 85-90% of patients! Hairy cell leukemia is one of the B-cell leukemias like CLL. It only comprises about 2% of leukemias but make sure you can recognize a "hairy" cell on smear for the exam.

363. Answer: D

The correct answer is proceed with combination chemotherapy without laparotomy. This patient has Stage IIIB Hodgkin's disease. Further workup is not needed as the CT scan indicated disease on both sides of the diaphragm. Additionally he has "B" symptoms with night sweats. Treatment should proceed with combination chemotherapy. Further surgery or workup is not indicated at this time.

364. Answer: A

The correct answer is >75% are B-cell lymphomas. This seems to be a question of the ABIM that they traditionally ask. Why? I don't know..but KNOW that most non-Hodgkin's lymphomas are B-Cell type. Follicular lymphomas are usually quite INDOLENT. Burkitt's lymphoma is a type of non-Hodgkin's lymphoma and the African-form is associated with Epstein-Barr virus infection.

365. Answer: E

The correct answer is the lytic lesions on plain films would NOT "light up" on the bone scan. This patient has multiple myeloma most likely. Multiple myeloma cells produce osteoclast activating factor, which induces the osteoclast to form lytic bone lesions WITHOUT new bone formation. New bone formation is required for "lighting up" on the bone scan. It is unlikely that this patient would have osteomyelitis because of his multiple myeloma. Neither renal failure nor Rouleaux formation would be contraindications for bone scan.

366. Answer: C

The correct answer is vigorous hydration with normal saline with furosemide to maintain urine output at 200cc/hour followed by biphosphonate pamidronate. The best treatment is to hydrate the patient aggressively and then use furosemide to increase urinary excretion of calcium. Biphosphonate pamidronate will not work acutely but will begin to work in the first 24 hours to help provide prolonged response. A volume expander is required like normal saline and not free water like ¼ normal saline.

367. Answer: B

The correct answer is if the genital warts are due to Human Papillomavirus type 16 or 18. The way I remember this is that kids get their driver's license in most states at age 16 and can vote at age 18—(both of these are potentially bad things depending on the habits of the 16 and 18 year old). These types are thought to express an E7 protein which binds to the retinoblastoma protein inactivating the retinoblastoma tumor-suppressor gene. Types 31 and 35 have also been implicated. I don't have any good pneumonics for 31 and 35 except that some view 31 as a "bad age" as you are now in your 30s for sure and 35 is really bad cause you are ½ way to 40. (sorry not much help on these 2).

368. Answer: C

The correct answer is combination pelvic irradiation and chemotherapy. She has regional lymph node involvement without metastasis = Duke's C so chemotherapy is indicated. She has rectal carcinoma too and so radiation therapy is helpful in this context.

369. Answer: B

The correct answer is to do a Bone Scan. This is the first staging test done in the workup of Prostate Cancer. If abnormalities are found on the bone scan you then proceed to do plain-film x-rays of the areas to exclude other possible causes. Then you would do surgical staging with removal and examination of the surrounding nodes (often done with prostatectomy).

370. Answer: A

The correct answer is 95%. With a seminoma and confined to the testes (Stage I) there is a 95% survival rate with radiation therapy. This is one of the most curable types of cancer especially if treated and recognized early.

371. Answer: D

The correct answer is modified radical mastectomy and tamoxifen for 5 years. The lesion is >4cm—therefore she should get a radical mastectomy. She is postmenopausal so you must look at her Hormone receptor (HR) status to determine what to do next: If it is positive: she gets only tamoxifen; if it is Negative she only gets chemotherapy.

372. Answer: B

The correct answer is modified radical mastectomy with chemotherapy and tamoxifen for 5 years. The lesion is >4cm—therefore she should get a radical mastectomy. She is premenopausal so she automatically gets chemotherapy. Finally you need to know the hormonal status to determine if she should get tamoxifen; if it is positive: she gets tamoxifen; if it is negative she only gets chemotherapy and no tamoxifen.

373. Answer: E

The correct answer is oral contraceptive use is NOT associated with increased risk of ovarian cancer and actually will decrease risk. BRCA1 (17q21) is associated with a 40% lifetime risk of developing ovarian cancer and accounts for most patients with familial ovarian cancer. BRCA2 (13q12-13) is associated with a 10-20% risk of ovarian cancer. Nulliparity and a positive family history also both increase risk but to a lesser extent.

374. Answer: A

The correct answer is multiple myeloma. This elderly patient has bone pain, hypercalcemia and anemia. His x-ray shows osteoporosis and he has a negative bone scan. The best fit for a diagnosis would be multiple myeloma. Myeloma can cause diffuse osteoporosis as well as anemia and hypercalcemia. An important pearl about myeloma is that bone lesions do not show up on bone scan. Metastatic prostate or lung cancer would likely show up on bone scan. Prolonged steroid use and avascular necrosis would not cause hypercalcemia and anemia.

375. Answer: A

The correct answer is Breast Cancer. Unfortunately even with physical examination of the breast combined with mammogram, a good number of breast cancers will be undiagnosed before they disseminate.

376. Answer: B

The correct answer is metastatic germ cell tumor of the testis. The findings of endocrine abnormalities (gynecomastia) as initial presentation support a germ cell tumor as well as the now enlarged testis (which may not have been present at the time of initial diagnosis). Pulmonary metastases with germ cell tumor of the testis is common.

377. Answer: E

The correct answer is doxorubicin (Adriamycin). It is NOT associated with peripheral neuropathy.

378. Answer: C

The correct answer is head and neck cancer.

379. Answer: D

The correct answer is small cell carcinoma of the lung. Remember "small cells" do a lot of stuff—SIADH, Ectopic ACTH production, and Eaton-Lambert (myasthenic) syndrome.

380. Answer: A

The correct answer is ovarian cancer. Not a lot of explanation here—sorry. This is pretty straightforward just memorize it.

381. Answer: A

The correct answer is CT scan without contrast. This patient has symptoms consistent with acute subarachnoid hemorrhage. He is at the average age for this to occur (45), has sudden onset of a severe headache, and no prior history of severe headaches. The neck stiffness is due to meningeal irritation from blood. Blood in the subarachnoid space shows up very well on CT scan and contrast is NOT needed. Acute bleeds are better imaged by non-contrast CT scan than MRIs. The CT scan is a preferable first option over a lumbar puncture, because if the CT is positive, an LP would not be necessary.

382. Answer: E

The correct answer is no imaging. This patient has typical symptoms of migraine headaches. She is at a common age (22) for the onset of migraines. Migraines are more common in women. The quality standards subcommittee of the American Academy of Neurology does not recommend the use of CNS imaging in adult patients with recurrent headaches typical of migraine, without focal neurologic signs or symptoms.

383. Answer: D

The correct answer is Head MRI. This 31-year-old woman has recurrent neurologic symptoms, with improvement between episodes. This history is suggestive of multiple sclerosis (MS). The most sensitive imaging procedure for MS is MRI. Although lesions can occur in the spinal cord, the brain is the best first imaging site.

384. Answer: E

The correct answer is reaction to phenytoin. This patient is having a reaction to phenytoin, creating pseudolymphoma syndrome. He has fever, elevated transaminases, and generalized lymphadenopathy. A negative RPR effectively rules out secondary syphilis. He has no exposure history to suggest hepatitis B or tularemia. Hodgkin's disease is a possibility, but the rapid onset, involvement of the liver, and diffuse lymphadenopathy would indicate advanced disease, less likely for such a rapid presentation.

385. Answer: C

The correct answer is stop tramadol. This older patient is evaluated for seizure. You are given the information that he has a negative contrast head CT scan (this makes tumor as a cause very unlikely). He is on a medication that has been associated with seizures (tramadol-trade name Ultram). This medication should be stopped and the patient should have further evaluation only if he has additional seizures off this medication.

386. Answer: E

The correct answer is none of the choices are likely. This patient has had headaches for six months. The most likely diagnosis is headache associated with oral contraceptive pills. She has a small risk for pseudotumor cerebri since she is obese. This diagnosis is excluded by the normal funduscopic exam. There are no cutaneous features suggestive of tuberous sclerosis (ash leaf spot, adenoma sebaceum).

387. Answer: E

The correct answer is gabapentin. This elderly patient is suffering from postherpetic neuralgia. Because of his history of coronary artery disease and BPH, tricyclic antidepressants (amitriptyline and nortriptyline) would be contraindicated. In patients with BPH, tricyclics can cause acute urinary retention. There is a higher risk for arrhythmia in patients with CAD treated with TCA. Gabapentin is effective and well tolerated for the treatment of post-herpetic neuralgia. Narcotics can be used for treatment of post-herpetic neuralgia, but a long-acting narcotic like OxyContin would not be the first option. Narcotics are more toxic in the elderly and in this case could lead to urinary retention. The anti-seizure medications gabapentin (Neurontin) and carbamazepine (Tegretol) are effective for post-herpetic neuralgia. Phenytoin (Dilantin) is not usually used because of toxicity and unproven efficacy.

388. Answer: D

The correct answer is multiple sensory deficits. This elderly patient notices disequilibrium when she walks. The key information is that her symptoms are improved when she touches a wall. She does not have vertigo symptoms. If she had orthostatic hypotension, her symptoms would not improve with touching a wall. Both benign positional vertigo and vestibular neuronitis have symptoms of vertigo, which this patient does not have. She is elderly, which is the population multiple sensory deficits are seen in. These patients may have visual, hearing, orthopedic, and neuropathy problems. The sum total of these sensory problems makes the patient feel unsteady. When sensory input from the hand (touching the wall) is included, she feels more stable.

389. Answer: A

The correct answer is Nylen-Bárány maneuver. This patient has very brief episodes of vertigo, which usually occur when he has a sudden change of position such as rolling over in bed. This is the classic description of benign positional vertigo. This diagnosis is confirmed clinically with the Nylen-Bárány maneuver (also called the Hallpike-Dix maneuver). There is no specific testing such as an audiogram ENG or MRI that would make this diagnosis.

390. Answer: D

The correct answer is cerumen impaction. This patient has noticed decreased hearing in his right ear. He has risk factors for hearing loss, including recent treatment with aminoglycosides. The results of the Rinne test and Weber test are diagnostic in this case. The Rinne test shows air conduction louder than bone conduction in the left ear and bone conduction louder than air conduction in the right ear (symptomatic ear). This is consistent with a conductive hearing loss in his right ear. The Weber test confirms this bilateralizing to the ear with the conductive hearing loss. Aminoglycoside toxicity would cause a sensory hearing loss, as would acoustic neuroma and Ménière's disease and cochlear osteosclerosis. Unilateral cerumen impaction would cause a conductive hearing loss on the side of the impaction.

391. Answer: A

The correct answer is have the patient call 911 for emergency evaluation/transport to ER. This patient has symptoms consistent with CO poisoning: headache, nausea, vomiting, diarrhea, and dyspnea. The key piece of clinical information is the improvement when he went outside to shovel snow. The appropriate management would be immediate removal from his home and immediate supportive care in an ER.

392. Answer: B

The correct answer is seizure (post-ictal). When confronted with a question like this, narrow the list first. Stroke is unlikely because of his age and the lack of focal neurologic findings. Encephalitis is unlikely without a fever and elevated white count. Hyperglycemia is out – the routine labs are negative. Drug intoxication is possible, as is a seizure/post-ictal state. Of these choices, seizure wins over drug intoxications because of the lack of findings on examination (no papillary abnormalities).

393. Answer: C

The correct answer is toxicology. Although several of the tests would probably be performed while the patient is in the ED, the Boards are looking for *a single, best answer*. Given that there is no evidence of trauma, and no focal neurological deficits, the CT and skull x-ray are unlikely to help. The lack of meningeal signs eliminates diagnoses like encephalitis and subarachnoid hemorrhage, so the lumbar puncture is less likely to help. An ABG might help if carbon monoxide (CO) poisoning were suspected; however, we are told that his apartment was well ventilated. Also, CO poisoning occurs most often in older persons who use petroleum-burning space heaters in the winter. Although we see no evidence of drug intoxication on exam, toxicology would be very helpful in this situation. Also if you did question 392 before this one—you might be angry—"But, but drug intoxication is not what this guy had last question!!" Here is the rub—on the ABIM—always look for the BEST POSSIBLE ANSWER of the choices. Sometimes depending on the responses given, you will get several responses that "look" good however, always seek out the "BEST" choice of what is listed.

394. Answer: C

The correct answer is cluster headache. The normal exam in combination with these symptoms describes a cluster headache. For the exam, you must know the difference between each of the listed headaches.

395. Answer: E

The correct answer is that all of the choices are correct. All of the listed agents are effective in treating cluster headaches.

396. Answer: B

The correct answer is abscess. In this case, the gradually worsening headaches after an invasive procedure strongly suggest an abscess. The fever and focal neurological deficits confirm this. Remember, the triad of fever, focal deficits, and headache means *abscess*. In bacterial meningitis, there are usually no focal neurological deficits.

397. Answer: D

The correct answer is Ménière's disease. The triad of episodic vertigo, hearing loss, and tinnitus makes this the most likely diagnosis. In benign positional vertigo, the person would not be expected to have hearing loss. Labyrinthitis and neuronitis are usually monophasic illnesses, likely due to a virus. Although stroke can cause vertigo, it is unlikely to be recurrent. In addition, stroke rarely causes vertigo by itself.

398. Answer: A

The correct answer is cerebellar infarct. Infarct is most likely to explain the sudden onset of this constellation of signs and symptoms. Cerebellar infarct is very dangerous, and anyone with this diagnosis should be observed closely. As swelling occurs, there is a risk of compression of the brainstem. If the brainstem is at risk, surgery may be necessary as a life-saving procedure.

399. Answer: A

The correct answer is subarachnoid hemorrhage. The sequence of events is critical to the diagnosis. The headache was sudden: "Thunder-clap," and "Worst headache of my life" are common descriptors. It is not unusual for a person to lose consciousness with a subarachnoid bleed. Often, they appear better following this, and then worsen. The sign that shows meningeal irritation is meningismus. A low-grade fever is common. A stroke would not cause meningismus. Herpes is usually slower in onset, and associated with a high fever. Often, herpes causes changes in mentation prior to other symptoms. Abscesses and tumors are more likely to cause focal neurological deficits.

400. Answer: B

The correct answer is multiple sclerosis. The most likely diagnosis is multiple sclerosis (MS). The history of transient neurologic dysfunction (the blurred vision in college) strongly supports the diagnosis. The patient has an upper motor neuron disease (the increased reflexes and positive Babinski), so Cauda Equina syndrome and Guillain-Barré are not possible. The symptoms only involve the left side, so transverse myelitis, which would cause a paraparesis, is not possible. Stroke is unlikely because the patient is young, without risk factors for stroke, and the symptoms have gradually worsened for ten days. She denies orthostatic hypotension.

401. Answer: B

The correct answer is Parkinson's disease. Since he is on no medications, he does not have a drug-induced Parkinsonism (not a choice here). Shy-Drager by definition includes severe orthostasis. Striatonigral degeneration looks like Parkinson's without the resting tremor. PSP includes loss of voluntary vertical gaze and axial rigidity (more than appendicular). PSP is also highly associated with dementia. Alzheimer's and

Parkinson's can overlap; however, Alzheimer's does not begin with these symptoms, and is therefore very unlikely.

---

402. Answer: E

The correct answer is Tensilon test. This patient has a characteristic presentation of Myasthenia Gravis. The age of onset is between the second and fourth decades of life. Myasthenia is due to circulating polyclonal IgG autoantibodies (produced by B-lymphocytes) to the acetylcholine receptor. It is characterized by weakness that worsens with physical activity. In about 40% of cases, the presenting complaint is diplopia. Other common symptoms include dysarthria, dysphagia, and decreased range of facial movements. Limb and neck weakness is common. It is uncommon for the limbs to be affected without other symptoms. Medications such as D-penicillamine (once used to treat rheumatoid arthritis) can cause drug-induced myasthenia. If the drug is discontinued, the myasthenia-like syndrome resolves. Although TIA and stroke must be considered in the diagnosis, it is very unusual for ischemia to produce diplopia alone. Often, other neurological symptoms are present. Graves ophthalmopathy must always be considered when a patient has diplopia. Often, physical signs of Graves' disease, such as the Graves' stare, will suggest a diagnosis of thyroid disease.

The first diagnostic test is the Tensilon test. When clinical signs are present (not just subjective diplopia), the Tensilon test can confirm the clinical diagnosis. Tensilon (edrophonium) is a short-acting acetylcholinesterase inhibitor that acts to prolong the effects of acetylcholine at the postsynaptic neuromuscular junction. This will reverse the weakness transiently. A positive test, then, would be improvement in clinical signs. A second test is the acetylcholine receptor antibody test. It is positive in 50% of patients with ocular myasthenia, and positive in 90% of patients with generalized myasthenia. In this case (ocular symptoms only), it would be a second line test. CT of the chest would be indicated to eliminate the possibility of a thymoma, which is present in about 15% of patients with Myasthenia Gravis. EMG may be performed as a confirmatory test as well. The classic EMG finding in Myasthenia Gravis is the electrodecremental response to repetitive stimulation. An MRI of the brain would not be needed.

---

403. Answer: D

The correct answer is adult-onset Still's disease. The combination of a rash and joint pain in an adult should always alert one to the possibility of adult-onset Still's. The patients often have fevers, high white counts, and a high Sed rate. Even though the patient is ANA positive, there is nothing to suggest lupus.

---

404. Answer: A

The correct answer is Sjögren's syndrome with non-Hodgkin's lymphoma. The patient obviously has Sjögren's syndrome. The lymph nodes sound ominous in description and there is a significantly increased relative risk of non-Hodgkin's lymphoma in patients with Sjögren's syndrome. In general, there is a higher risk of non-Hodgkin's lymphoma with most of the connective tissue disease processes.

---

405. Answer: C

The correct answer is anti-histone antibody. Anti-SCL70 is found in 8% of scleroderma patients. ANAs are frequently found in patients with scleroderma. Anti-centromere antibody is often found with CREST syndrome. Rheumatoid factors are nonspecific in this situation, but anti-histone antibodies are usually found in drug-induced lupus.

406. Answer: B

The correct answer is gout. She has myeloma and osteoarthritis. She has a fairly typical presentation of gout in the setting of a non-benign disease. The unusual feature is that her gouty attack is taking place in her Heberden's node.

407. Answer: E

The correct answer is prednisone 15 mg/day. Her symptoms are typical of polymyalgia rheumatica. One would only use 60 mg of prednisone if there was any evidence of giant cell arteritis.

408. Answer: B

The correct answer is physical therapy. The patient has several risk factors for frozen shoulder syndrome and the appropriate treatment is aggressive physical therapy. Perhaps non-steroidals could be used but physical therapy is the first option.

409. Answer: C

The correct answer is CT scan of joints. The patient has a seronegative spondyloarthropathy and is likely to be HLA B-27 positive. CT scan of the SI joints is very useful for showing bony erosive changes.

410. Answer: A

The correct "incorrect" answer is prednisone 10 mg. The patient seems to have clinical evidence suggestive of carpal tunnel entrapment. Release, splint, and corticosteroid injection are all appropriate, but not prednisone by mouth.

411. Answer: B

The correct answer is rapidly progressive GN with crescents. This patient clearly has Wegener's granulomatosis. With the proliferative sediment and the rapid increase in creatinine, RPGN is the likely diagnosis.

412. Answer: E

The correct answer is sputum for AFB. The anti-TNF drugs have been associated with a higher risk of TB.

413. Answer: A

The correct answer is positive anti-centromere antibodies. She has had stable Raynaud's for ten years. Therefore, to suddenly now develop a connective tissue disease process is unlikely. The dilated capillaries are of concern. ANA's are found in 20% of patients with primary Raynaud's. Anti-centromere is seen in CREST.

414. Answer: C

The correct answer is occasional ECHO to estimate pulmonary pressure. This patient has CREST syndrome. While the prognosis is generally regarded as one of the more benign variants of scleroderma, nevertheless, pulmonary HTN unrelated to pulmonary involvement is well described. Therefore, it would be important to look for the early presence of pulmonary HTN, particularly given the newer groups of medications that could potentially arrest this.

415. Answer: A

The correct "incorrect" answer is IV immunoglobulin. This patient obviously has dermatomyositis and will require long-term corticosteroid therapy. Therefore, according to the latest recommendations of the American College of Rheumatology, any patient requiring prednisone at a dose of 5 mg, qd. or greater for a period of three months or longer will require a bisphosphonate. Bone loss is dramatic in the first few weeks after initiating glucocorticoids, particularly at higher doses. However, dramatic bone loss occurs even at a relatively low dose of 7.5 mg, qd.

416. Answer: C

The correct answer is diabetic-limited joint mobility syndrome. This lady has classic features of diabetic-limited joint mobility syndrome to include a positive prayer's sign, history of presumed "frozen shoulder syndrome," Dupuytren's contractures and carpal tunnel syndrome. She has pseudo-scleroderma of Buschke. Other features include rotator cuff tendinitis, rotator cuff calcification, and bicipital tendinitis. If the stenosing tenosynovitis is caught early, which is responsible for her triggering, then a local corticosteroid injection is highly appropriate. Of course, there may be a temporary loss of diabetic control. However, if the stenosis of her tendon sheaths is fairly chronic, then a simple operative procedure by a hand surgeon would be appropriate.

417. Answer: B

The correct answer is non-caseating granulomatous inflammatory changes. She has multi-organ involvement to suggest the diagnosis of sarcoidosis. The initial lesions on her legs were probably those of erythema nodosum. A biopsy would have found a probable panniculitis. Hyper-calcemia, facial nerve palsy and cutaneous involvement is, again, typical. ACE levels may be elevated, but not always. A chest x-ray would probably be appropriate as part of her work-up.

418. Answer: D

The correct answer is repeat ANA, anti-dsDNA titers, anti-centromere, and anti-SCL70. The patient most likely has primary Raynaud's. Approximately 20% of younger women with primary Raynaud's have a positive ANA and this is not always an appropriate screening test. However, given the fact that her ANA is known to be positive, it would be appropriate and reassuring to exclude a secondary process. Her symptoms do not particularly suggest a connective tissue disease process, but a repeat ANA would be appropriate because of variations from lab to lab. The specific serologies for lupus including anti-dsDNA and SM would be reasonable. So, too, would be an anti-centromere to rule out CREST and an anti-SCL70 to exclude scleroderma. If these last two tests were found to be positive, then a further screening to include manometry, ECHO, etc., would be appropriate. The negative vital capillaroscopy is indeed reassuring.

419. Answer: C

The correct answer is check baseline labs to include CBC, Sed rate, RF and aspirate one of the knees. This patient has a classic reactive arthritis, probably acquired through a GI route. She provides no history to suggest any other reactive features to include urethritis or conjunctivitis. IV antibiotics would obviously have been inappropriate. It would be more appropriate to aspirate the joint and have baseline labs checked before proceeding to systemic corticosteroids or local joint injection.

420. Answer: E

The correct "incorrect" answer is prednisone 10 mg, qd. This patient is elderly and has had a previous history of peptic ulcer and, therefore, is classically at risk for life-threatening GI bleed. The coxibs have been developed specifically for this purpose and there are outcome studies to demonstrate a significant reduction in life-threatening bleeds in two of the mentioned drugs. Hydrocodone is obviously addictive and is the last option for this patient. There is no reason to give him systemic corticosteroid therapy.

421. Answer: A

The correct answer is MRI of the LS-spine. This patient has classic symptoms of inflammatory back pain, suggesting sacroiliitis. An MRI would be very expensive and inappropriate. While early changes may be missed on a simple film of the LS-spine and SI joints, a CT scan is highly sensitive for erosive changes in the SI joints and would be most appropriate. Sub-clinical uveitis needs to be excluded in this patient. His GI symptoms certainly may suggest that he has inflammatory bowel disease, which certainly could be related to his musculoskeletal symptoms.

422. Answer: B

The correct answer is alendronate 70 mg, q week or risedronate 30 mg, q week. She has PMR. Any patient who is going to be on prednisone at a dose of 5 mg, q.d. for longer than three months should be placed on a bisphosphonate as prophylaxis against glucocorticoid-induced osteoporosis with potential for fractures. She has polymyalgia rheumatica and the average patient requires glucocorticoid therapy for about one year. These are current recommendations of the American College of Rheumatology. SERMs have not clinically been demonstrated to have this effect.

423. Answer: B

The correct answer is ferritin and calcium levels. This patient presumably has calcium pyrophosphate deposition disease (CPPD). He should be instructed to come in and have his joints aspirated during an acute flare. Positively birefringent crystals will probably be aspirated at that time. In the interim, hemochromatosis and hyperparathyroidism, the two very strong associations with CPPD, need to be excluded.

424. Answer: D

The correct answer is dermatomyositis. Note that he has "Gottron papules" on his knuckles, which is the most specific finding for this disorder. The elevated aldolase is helpful as well as the proximal muscle weakness. Remember the stupid ANA is non-specific in the speckled pattern. Another classic finding that he doesn't have is the "heliotrope" rash on the upper eyelids.

425. Answer: C

The correct answer is impingement syndrome. This refers to compression of the subacromial bursa or regional tendons in the space between the acromion and the humeral head. The biceps tendon and all the rotator cuff tendons go through this area. The passive abduction to 90 degrees causing pain in the deltoid region is the test that nails this one. A rotator cuff tear would cause more pain during active abduction than passive abduction. Bursitis of the subacromial bursa would do the same thing. Osteoarthritis of the shoulder is very rare. A thoracic outlet syndrome would cause pain that extends from the base of the neck, over the top of the shoulder, and down the arm.

426. Answer: A

The correct answer is *Mycobacterium marinum*. Note that he has a chronic process x 2 years. It is associated with water. Put the two together and you come up with *Mycobacterium marinum*! Note it is not unusual for you NOT to be able to culture this organism. Again, the water exposure is the kicker here. Think of the other organisms if the environmental exposure is right: *Nocardia*—soil; *Blastomyces*—soil or lumber; *Sporothrix*—gardens or plants.

427. Answer: E

The correct answer is hepatitis C serology. This patient has cryoglobulinemia. It is mixed due to the abnormally high rheumatoid factor binding to either monoclonal or polyclonal IgG. Vasculitis with purpura is the most common presentation for mixed cryoglobulinemia. Hepatitis C has a very strong association with mixed cryoglobulinemia! In one study, 86% of cryoglobulinemics were positive for hepatitis C!! The monoclonal type is due to multiple myeloma or Waldenström's macroglobulinemia—with this you would expect to see severe hemolytic anemia and something in the history like Raynaud's or cyanosis with exposure to cold.

428. Answer: B

The correct answer is avascular necrosis of the hip. Up to 1/3 of SLE patients on chronic steroids will develop avascular necrosis of a hip. Best way to diagnose it is with an MRI. The acute onset makes you steer away from the osteomyelitis area. A fracture should have been seen on plain film.

429. Answer: B

The correct answer is dual-energy x-ray absorptiometry (DEXA). This is the newest and cheapest method. It is also the quickest. Precision of the DEXA approaches 1-2%. The quantitative CT scan and dual photon absorptiometry take a lot of time. The CT scan also gives a lot of radiation.

430. Answer: D

The correct answer is loss of lower esophageal sphincter function. Note that this is the most common abnormality seen. However, for those of you who went for the diverticulum—yes, if you saw that it is pathognomonic, BUT it is rarer than loss of the lower esophageal sphincter tone…a trick question...but sometimes the mean old ABIM can be tricky too.

431. Answer: C

The correct answer is Behçet's syndrome. Behçet's syndrome is a recurrent disease of unknown etiology and is characterized by painful oral and genital ulcers, eye inflammation, arthritis, and CNS symptoms with fever and abdominal complaints. Thrombophlebitis can also occur with this syndrome. This can mimic inflammatory bowel disease by the CNS symptoms (headache), so steer away from this. Whipple's disease is associated with arthritis, abdominal pain, and CNS disease, but NOT the aphthous ulcers or thrombophlebitis.

432. Answer: C

The correct answer to this question is allopurinol—which you would NOT use for treatment of acute gouty arthritis! The nonsteroidal anti-inflammatory drugs, either form of colchicine, or the intraarticular steroids can be used in the acute presentation. Colchicine inhibits neutrophil activation by inhibiting crystal-induced protein tyrosine phosphorylation. Many patients, because of the GI side effects, do not tolerate oral colchicine. Colchicine may be given IV, but administration by this route is dangerous and you have to be careful. You can't use IV colchicine in the face of bone marrow dysfunction, renal/liver disease, or sepsis. Allopurinol, remember, will PROLONG the attack so it should definitely be avoided!

433. Answer: E

The correct answer is pseudogout. Calcium pyrophosphate dihydrate (CPPD) crystals cause chondrocalcinosis (calcium in the cartilage). Pseudogout is the term used for the acute presentation of the disease. The crystals of pseudogout have weakly positive birefringence on compensated polarized light microscopy as opposed to gout where the crystals have strongly negative birefringence under polarized light. KNOW THIS!! And look at pictures of these two and be able to discern between them. Pictures are in the Forbes and Jackson's Clinical Pocket Guide included with the Core. If you don't have this—go to the Internet and search under Google or whatever search engine you like and look for "picture of calcium pyrophosphate dihydrate crystals"—you'll find a picture really fast.

434. Answer: A

The correct answer is Reiter's syndrome. Reiter's syndrome is a classic form of reactive arthritis in which there occurs a triad of nonspecific urethritis, conjunctivitis, and asymmetric arthritis. The arthritis usually involves the large joint of the lower extremities. Causes of Reiter's syndrome and other reactive arthritis are genitourinary infections from *Chlamydia* or *Ureaplasma* and gastrointestinal infections due to *Salmonella, Shigella, Yersinia, Klebsiella, and Campylobacter.*

435. Answer: D

The correct answer is Raynaud's phenomenon. This is NOT used as a manifestation to diagnose lupus erythematosus. BE SURE you know the 11 diagnostic criteria mentioned in the Rheumatology text. They will give you a patient with non-specific findings and you will have to know to find 4 or more of the 11 to diagnose SLE. The 11 are: photosensitivity, blood changes (anemia, leukopenia, etc.), renal disease, +ANA, +anti-dsDNA or anti-Sm antibody, arthritis, malar rash, discoid rash, neuropsychiatric features (psychosis, seizures), oral lesions, and serositis.

436. Answer: B

The correct answer is Heberden's node. This is NOT seen in rheumatoid arthritis but is seen in osteoarthritis. All of the other findings are consistent with long-standing Rheumatoid arthritis.

437. Answer: A

The correct answer is dsDNA antibody. As active as her disease is, it would be good to check and see if she is dsDNA antibody positive. This would confirm the diagnosis of SLE. Her renal involvement in particular should correlate with presence of dsDNA antibody also. The anti-SM antibody is much less likely to be positive. The RNP antibody is mainly seen with mixed connective tissue disease, but can be found in SLE on occasion. The SS-A (Ro) antibody is more helpful with neonatal lupus, Sjögren's syndrome, and systemic sclerosis. Anti-histone is used to differentiate drug-induced lupus.

438. Answer: E

The correct answer is x-rays of the sacroiliac joints are indicated. This man has ankylosing spondylitis, at least based on his history and physical examination. The x-ray will show sacroiliitis with eventual fusion of the sacroiliac joint. The diagnosis must be differentiated from inflammatory bowel disease or psoriasis, which can give you similar findings as far as the arthropathy and sacroiliitis.

439. Answer: C

The correct answer is gout. His x-ray finds are consistent with long-standing gout and remember that the 1st metatarsophalangeal joint is the most common joint to be involved. Also he has chronic tophaceous gout with the findings of the tophaceous deposits of monosodium urate at his olecranon bursae. The other sites for these are the Achilles tendons and the external ear. Tophi are painless, but their presence in and around joints can limit joint mobility.

440. Answer: B

The correct answer is tell her that her risk of osteoporosis is very low and no testing is required at this time. She is menstruating and does not smoke. She exercises on a regular basis. She eats a normal diet. She is not of thin build. You could recommend calcium supplements to her as a prevention method before menopause develops. None of the other tests are needed at this point.

441. Answer: A

The correct answer is chronic oral steroid use. With his asthma history you have to wonder if he is not on chronic steroids. This will induce early osteoporosis especially in men. The other drugs listed are not associated with early osteoporosis.

442. Answer: C

The correct answer is corticosteroid injection into the carpal tunnel. You should at least try this before sending her to surgery for carpal tunnel release. The other choices are not indicated. Repeating the EMG/NCS would not help at this point.

443. Answer: B

The correct answer is exertional chest pain relieved with rest is NOT associated with osteoporosis. Obviously this woman is having pain, which must make you think about angina or coronary disease syndromes. All of the other findings are seen with osteoporosis. The pulmonary dysfunction can occur as the total lung capacity is reduced by changes in the architecture of the thorax due to disease progression and worsening dorsal kyphosis and cervical lordosis.

444. Answer: D

The correct answer is cyclosporine. This patient has typical clinical features of gout: acute onset of severe foot pain. He is on cyclosporine, a drug that increases uric acid levels and frequently can cause gout. Although aspirin in low doses can slightly increase gout risk, cyclosporine is much more likely (up to 30% develop gout). Alcohol can also increase the risk of gout, but no history of alcohol use is given in this case.

445. Answer: E

The correct answer is adverse effect due to ciprofloxacin. This patient develops Achilles tendon pain after a ski vacation. An acute injury from skiing is a possibility, but in the setting of prolonged ciprofloxacin use, quinolone-induced tendonitis/tendon injury is more likely. Tendon rupture related to quinolone use has been well documented in the literature with the most cases being attributed to ciprofloxacin. It is a side effect of the drug class and not related to any drug interactions.

446. Answer: B

The correct answer is acute hypersensitivity pneumonitis. Given the temporal relationship between his exposure to the mice, the nonspecific infiltrates, and the restrictive pulmonary physiology, this is the best answer listed. The best therapy is to remove him from this environment if at all possible, as chronic exposure could lead to a subacute or chronic form of this disease with potentially serious physiologic consequences.

447. Answer: E

The correct answer is to prescribe a metered dose albuterol inhaler before she exercises. Exercise-induced asthma can frequently be prevented by use of an inhaler shortly before the exercise event. The other agents would not be helpful in a preventative mode if used just before the exercise event. Since her symptoms are predictable, it is not necessary to subject her to prolonged medications for a majority of the time when she will not have any symptoms. (As an aside: Of course, earplugs may be effective if the music and man she is listening to is inducing the attack. If I had to exercise to that I likely would become ill too.)

448. Answer: C

The correct answer is cytoplasmic μ chains—the heavy chain of immunoglobulin M. Pre-B cells lack any membrane-bound immunoglobulin.

449. Answer: A

The correct answer is C1 esterase inhibitor. The classical pathway of complement activation is initiated by an antibody-antigen interaction. The first complement component is C1—a complex composed of 3 proteins. C1 binds to immune complexes with activation mediated by C1q. Active C1 then initiates the cleavage and concomitant activation of C4 and C2. A plasma protease inhibitor known as C1 esterase inhibitor destroys the activated C1. Patients like Mr. Dude may develop angioedema. It is usually an autosomal disorder but can be acquired in some malignant and autoimmune diseases. Danazol is very helpful in treating this disorder, as it will increase the level of C1 esterase inhibitor.

450. Answer: D

The correct answer is skin biopsy. The combination of residual skin lesions, arthralgias, and elevated ESR are not consistent with hereditary angioedema or most urticarial diseases. It is much more likely due to cutaneous necrotizing vasculitis, which could be confirmed by skin biopsy. Chronic urticaria is rarely allergic in nature; therefore, allergy skin testing and IgE levels are not likely to be helpful. C1 esterase inhibitor activity level would be useful in hereditary angioedema, but not in this entity. The patch test would be helpful in diagnosing contact dermatitis.

451. Answer: E

The correct answer is monocyte-derived IL-6 activation of T cells. Yes, they might ask you this. I mean, why not? They have tons of TB questions on the ABIM, so why not ask about the simplest test done to confirm infection with tuberculosis? Reactions are initiated by mononuclear white cells and require 48-72 hours to respond to an antigen exposure. This is a delayed-type hypersensitivity reaction. T cells and macrophages mediate the cellular events resulting in such hypersensitivity responses. Antigen is processed by monocytes/macrophages and presented to specific T cells. Macrophages will then secrete interleukin 1 and interleukin 6 to amplify the specific T cells and secrete interleukin 2 and interferon-gamma to bring in additional T cells and macrophages to join the inflammatory process. Macrophages brought in may undergo epithelioid cell transformation and form giant cells. All this put together results in the induration that we measure as a positive skin test! The main thing to remember is that the initial response is due to the mononuclear leukocytes as they activate T cells with IL-6.

452. Answer: B

The correct answer is monthly intravenous immunoglobulin. She has common variable immunodeficiency. B-cells can recognize antigen and multiply, but fail to differentiate to the immunoglobulin-secreting stage. Nodular lymphoid hyperplasia and splenomegaly is usually found in these patients. These patients have PAN-hypogammaglobulinemia. Think about this disease in anyone who presents with chronic pulmonary infections, unexplained bronchiectasis (like Ms. Yellow), recurrent Giardia, and atrophic gastritis. The therapy for common variable immunodeficiency is replacement of immunoglobulin—mainly immunoglobulin G—with IVIG. You would like the level to reach 500 mg/dl.

453. Answer: C

The correct answer is that all of the answers listed in this question are correct. Okay, just know this bugger. This is one of those "just memorize and move on" questions.

454. Answer: A

The correct answer is ataxia-telangiectasia syndrome. This is an autosomal recessive disorder that is associated with abnormal thymic development. The progressive cerebellar ataxia and telangiectasias are obviously hallmarks for this disease. The gene responsible is located on chromosome 11 (dang, hopefully they aren't going to ask that!). The defect in the gene results in an inability to repair damaged DNA. I threw in the adenosine deaminase deficiency just to remind you that it is NOT associated with ataxia-telangiectasia syndrome, but is associated with severe combined immunodeficiency.

455. Answer: C

The correct answer is horse antithymocyte globulin. He has developed a serum sickness-like illness. All of his features are classic for severe reaction to an agent like this. Usually it occurs eight to thirteen days after receiving the therapy.

456. Answer: B

The correct answer is direct activation of mediator release from mast cells, basophils, or both. Radiocontrast media directly activates these cells to release the mediators of anaphylaxis. This is in contrast to anaphylaxis due to bee stings, foods, and heterologous serum (such as tetanus antitoxin), which is likely due to an IgE-mediated reaction against the offending protein. Anaphylaxis due to penicillin and other antibiotics is due to IgE recognition of protein-hapten conjugants. Finally, dialysis induces anaphylaxis with complement activation.

457. Answer: E

The correct answer is by causing an IgE-mediated reaction against proteins in the sting media. Anaphylaxis due to bee stings, foods, and heterologous serum (such as tetanus antitoxin) is likely due to an IgE-mediated reaction against the offending protein. In contrast (bad pun, sorry), radiocontrast media directly activates these cells to release the mediators of anaphylaxis. Anaphylaxis due to penicillin and other antibiotics is due to IgE recognition of protein-hapten conjugants. Finally, dialysis induces anaphylaxis with complement activation.

458. Answer: D

The correct answer is she had IgE recognition of protein-hapten conjugants. Anaphylaxis due to penicillin and other antibiotics is due to IgE recognition of protein-hapten conjugants. Anaphylaxis due to bee stings, foods, and heterologous serum (such as tetanus antitoxin) is likely due to an IgE-mediated reaction against the offending protein. In contrast (bad pun, sorry), radiocontrast media directly activates these cells to release the mediators of anaphylaxis. Finally, dialysis induces anaphylaxis with complement activation.

459. Answer: B

The correct answer is systemic mastocytosis. She has a syndrome characterized by mast cell infiltration of the skin (the small bumps that are itchy—known as urticaria pigmentosa), and gastrointestinal mucosa involvement. Usually the spleen and liver are also involved. The ulcer she developed is from histamine-mediated hypersecretion of gastric acid. You can confirm the diagnosis by measuring urine for histamine metabolites or by measuring increased levels of serum histamine or mast cell-derived neutral protease tryptase.

460. Answer: A

The correct answer is Henoch-Schönlein purpura (HSP). He has the classic findings of purpura that is confined to the buttocks and lower extremities. Additionally he has signs of gastrointestinal involvement as well as glomerulonephritis. Most of the time HSP is self-limiting, but occasionally it can progress to a chronic form.

461. Answer: D

The correct answer is they lack readily detectable immunoglobulin of ANY class on their membranes. Remember that detectable immunoglobulin is found on B-cells.

462. Answer: D

The correct answer is that all of the statements are true. I threw this one in just so you could remember all of the wonderful things that IgA does for us—and you might get tested on during the ABIM torture (er.....I mean testing) session. It is really quite under-appreciated compared to IgG—the most common immunoglobulin in SERUM and IgM—the principal immunoglobulin in the primary immune response.

463. Answer: A

The correct answer is isolated IgA deficiency. Isolated IgA deficiency is the most common immunodeficiency and has an incidence between 1:600 and 1:800. People with this disorder have a normal or reduced number of B cells with surface IgA, but have an overabundance of immature cells that express both IgA and IgM. The problem is that it appears that the cells cannot secrete IgA effectively. Thus, there is a reduced amount of serum as well as secretory IgA. About 30-40% of people with IgA deficiency have antibodies to IgA, thus if they get exposed to IgA (like in blood products or IVIG) they will anaphylax.

464. Answer: C

The correct answer is most immune complexes are removed by the reticuloendothelial system. Deposition of the immune complexes in tissues other than the reticuloendothelial system is what results in signs and symptoms of immune-complex disease. It appears that persistence of complexes is required for the development of renal disease. Immune complex-mediated vascular damage can lead to cutaneous necrotizing vasculitis.

465. Answer: A

The correct answer is mature red blood cells. All other cells of the body express Class I HLA antigens. Remember that Class I HLA antigens are encoded at the A, B, and C loci of the human major histocompatibility complex on chromosome 6. The Class I HLA antigens are useful in predicting results for organ transplants.

466. Answer: B

The correct answer is decongestant/nasal irrigation. This patient presents with a 5-day history of rhinorrhea, sore throat, and facial pain. She is afebrile with swollen nasal turbinates on exam. Her symptom complex is most consistent with the common cold. The CDC campaign to limit antibiotic use advises to wait 7-10 days before considering treatment with antibiotics for "sinusitis" for facial pain/persistent congestion. The yellow discharge does not increase the likelihood of a bacterial infection. The best treatment would be to begin saline nasal irrigation and topical decongestants for several days WITHOUT antibiotic treatment.

467. Answer: D

The correct answer is C1 esterase inhibitor. The classical pathway of complement activation is initiated by antibody-antigen interaction. The first complement component (C1, a complex composed of 3 proteins) binds to immune complexes with activation mediated by C1q. Active C1 then initiates the cleavage and concomitant activation of components C4 and C2. The activated C1 is destroyed by a plasma protease inhibitor known as C1 esterase inhibitor. Patients with deficiencies of C1 esterase inhibitor may develop angioedema, which can lead to death if it involves the larynx or other parts of the respiratory tract. Danazol therapy produces a great increase in the level and can alleviate the symptoms.

468. Answer: C

The correct response to this question is that anaphylactoid reactions are all of the choices EXCEPT that they are usually NOT immune responses. Anaphylactoid reactions are systemic reactions that have the same symptoms as anaphylaxis. They are NOT IgE-dependent and are usually NOT immune. Radiographic contrast agents and non-steroidal anti-inflammatory drugs are examples of these types of reactions.

469. Answer: E

The correct answer is that it is associated with a low IgM. Usually these patients have HIGH IgA and IgEs. They are at increased risk for infection and they can be treated successfully with bone marrow transplantation.

470. Answer: B

The correct answer is to give epinephrine 1/1000 0.5cc SQ. Expect at least one of these on the "real" test. Remember that IV steroids are not effective acutely. She is NOT hypotensive so she does not need epinephrine IV, and then you would use the 1/10,000 formulation of 5cc with fluid expanders and possibly dopamine if needed. Beta-blockage would be a disaster and you would not want to do that! It will blunt the effect of your epinephrine also! If she had bronchospasm you would consider aminophylline. Use of diphenhydramine and cimetidine is also helpful after the epinephrine.

471. Answer: B

The correct answer is to check for serum immunoglobulins. He most likely has immunoglobulin A deficiency. IgA serves as the first line of defense against infections of the respiratory tract as well as infections of the GI and GU tracts. IgA deficiency is really fairly common! 1/ 600 individuals of European ancestry will have the deficiency. People with IgA deficiency are usually healthy, but they may have frequent episodes of upper respiratory tract infections, bronchiectasis, and chronic diarrhea. They are also more prone to allergies, asthma, and other autoimmune disorders.

472. Answer: A

The correct answer is Kawasaki's disease. She has all of the classic findings: She has fever, which is a requirement, and then she has 1) conjunctivitis, 2) erythematous mouth and pharynx, strawberry tongue, and red, cracked lips, 3) a generalized rash, 4) changes to the peripheral extremities consisting of induration of the hands and feet with red palms and soles, and 5) a unilateral cervical lymph node enlarged to more than 1.5 cm in diameter. Patients have to have fever and at least 4 of the 5 findings. If there are less than 4 classic findings, then a diagnosis of atypical Kawasaki's should be considered. Treatment is with IVIG 2 grams/kg x 1 time dose over 12-14 hours and aspirin in high doses initially followed by low maintenance doses. Usually this occurs in children under the age of 5; however, cases in teenagers have been reported.

473. Answer: D

The correct answer is aspirin. All NSAIDS inhibit the synthesis of prostaglandins via binding to cyclooxygenase. However, aspirin is the ONLY agent that binds irreversibly. This is likely why aspirin is the only NSAID that inhibits platelets—platelets cannot manufacture new cyclooxygenase! Therefore, remember to stop aspirin 7-10 days before elective surgical procedures where bleeding cannot be tolerated (eye, neurosurgery, etc.)

474. Answer: C

The correct answer is topical tretinoin. The diagnosis of acne is established when three of the six lesions of acne are present. The lesions of acne are papules, pustules, open and closed comedones, ice pick scars, hyperpigmented macules, and cystic lesions. If, as in this patient, the majority of the lesions are non-inflammatory, topical retinoids are the treatment of choice because of their keratolytic effect. The other choices listed are not keratolytic, and thus would be less effective for the patient described.

475. Answer: B

The correct answer is that topical steroids do produce multiple side effects. Topical steroids had been the mainstay of therapy of treatment for atopic skin prior to the development of immune modulators, such as pimecrolimus and tacrolimus. Although both of the new drugs have local side effects, such as burning and stinging, topical steroids can cause striae, atrophy, telangiectasia, pigmentary changes, and acneform skin eruptions. Lubrication alone would not be expected to produce local side effects.

476. Answer: D

The correct answer is dermatomyositis and cancer. The classical presentation of dermatomyositis is a heliotrope rash about the eyes, proximal muscle weakness, erythema and telangiectasia of the cuticles, and palmar erythema. It is thought that the papules over the joints (Gottron's papules) are pathognomonic of dermatomyositis. Patients over 50 years of age are at risk for their dermatomyositis being associated with internal malignancy. The weight loss associated with the typical findings of dermatomyositis makes this the most likely diagnosis.

477. Answer: C

The correct answer is erythema nodosum. In addition to sarcoidosis, erythema nodosum can be associated with streptococcal infections, inflammatory bowel disease, tuberculosis, and drug allergy. The association of erythema nodosum, arthritis, anterior uveitis, and hilar adenopathy due to sarcoidosis is termed Lofgren's Syndrome, and is usually associated with a good prognosis. Although the classical Lofgren's syndrome is a tetrad, the term is commonly applied when a patient presents with only sarcoidosis and erythema nodosum. The lack of appropriate history and the appearance of the biopsy exclude the other diagnoses. Erythema nodosum can be treated with non-steroidal anti-inflammatory drugs, topical or systemic steroids, or immunosuppressive agents.

478. Answer: A

The correct answer is impetigo vulgaris. The trauma caused by scratching had broken the skin and permitted bacterial invasion and secondary infection. Most community-acquired skin infections are due to *Streptococcal* or *Staphylococcal* species. Impetigo vulgaris is most often caused by *Staphylococci*. Erythema nodosum most often presents as tender nodules on the pre-tibial surfaces of the legs. The diagnosis of acne vulgaris requires the presence of at least three of the six characteristic lesions. In general, drug eruptions most commonly start on the chest, abdomen, or the back.

479. Answer: D

The correct answer is bullous pemphigoid. Pemphigoid is a bullous disease of the elderly that may begin and remain on the legs for a number of years before involving the rest of the skin. It is pruritic in nature and can involve the mucosa. While occurring on normal or erythematous skin, the bullae give a negative Nikolsky's sign (which is positive in pemphigus). Grouped vesicles or urticarial lesions are more characteristic of dermatitis herpetiformis. The clinical appearance, history, and histology will rule out erythema multiforme. Direct immunofluorescence of skin adjacent to a bulla is positive with IgG and complement found in the lamina lucida of the basement membrane area. Because patients with pemphigoid have circulating antigens, indirect immunofluorescence is also frequently positive.

Treatment consists of topical steroids alone in localized disease, and systemic steroids, sulfones, tetracycline, and nicotinamide in widespread disease.

480. Answer: B

The correct answer is Hepatitis C. Hepatitis C is frequently found in association with PCT. In addition to vesicles of the skin, there can also be increased pigmentation, increased fragility, and milia formation. Patients with PCT also have an increased incidence of liver cirrhosis and liver cancer. Acanthosis nigricans and paraneoplastic pemphigus are not associated with PCT.

481. Answer: A

The correct answer is Herpetic infections. Exfoliative dermatitis is not associated with herpes simplex or *herpes zoster*. It is frequently seen as an allergic reaction to such drugs as sulfonamides, anti-malarials, penicillin, phenytoin, and barbiturates. It has also been associated with benign skin diseases such as atopic dermatitis, or malignant processes such as mycosis fungoides. Exfoliative dermatitis has also been found in association with solid tumors. No matter what the etiology, the skin biopsy is often non-specific. The course and prognosis of exfoliative dermatitis is related to the course of the underlying process.

482. Answer: C

The correct answer is glucagonoma syndrome. Erosions of the skin and mucous membranes characterize the Glucagonoma syndrome. The lesions are referred to as necrolytic migratory erythema. Patients may also have glossitis, weight loss, hyperglycemia, and decreased plasma amino acids. Sweet's syndrome (acute febrile neutrophilic dermatosis) presents with vesicular-like papules, fever, and leukocytosis. Carcinoid syndrome is characterized by flushing of the skin, and primary amyloidosis usually presents with pinch purpura.

When glucagonoma syndrome is diagnosed, it is important to rule out a zinc or magnesium deficiency because they can have a similar presentation. Patients with glucagonoma syndrome have an alpha cell tumor of the pancreas, and the sooner it is found and treated, the better the prognosis.

483. Answer: C

The correct answer is to refer her for excisional biopsy of the lesion. Superficial spreading melanoma is the most common type of melanoma, and comprises 70 percent of all melanomas. It is found predominately in young people who burn rather than tan. The favored location is on the back of the legs of women and on the backs of men. When such a lesion is identified, referral is indicated for simple excision and histological evaluation. Based on the depth of invasion, re-excision margins are decided and the patient's prognosis is determined. A punch biopsy of the brown area will show melanocytes in the epidermis, which may or may not be malignant and could result in an inaccurate diagnosis. Likewise, liquid nitrogen will only remove the superficial portion of the tumor, leaving the dermal portion to proliferate and metastasize. Whenever a melanoma is suspected, intervention is indicated because malignant melanoma is a life-threatening disease. By the year 2010 it is estimated that one in fifty people will have mclanoma.

484. Answer: D

The correct answer is sparfloxacin. This patient develops a rash after taking an antibiotic while on vacation in Hawaii. The distribution of the rash is strongly suggestive of a photosensitivity reaction. The quinolones have a varying phototoxicity profile, with sparfloxacin the most phototoxic. Norfloxacin is minimally phototoxic. Amoxicillin/clavulanate and nitrofurantoin do not cause phototoxic reactions.

485. Answer: E

The correct answer is cutaneous candidal infection. Typically these infections occur at sites that are chronically wet and macerated, such as an intertriginous area that requires frequent water exposure (like Ms. Times). Treatment would involve a topical agent such as topical clotrimazole.

486. Answer: B

The correct answer is dyshidrotic eczema. Hand dermatitis is quite common in individuals who wash their hands frequently, and Ms. Bulloch has a common variant of this. The finding of highly pruritic vesicles on the sides of the fingers is helpful in making this diagnosis. *Lichen planus* is a disorder with papulosquamous pruritic lesions that have a purplish hue. Zoster would present as a group of vesicles on an erythematous base. Atopic dermatitis would be more likely if she had a history of asthma or disease during childhood.

487. Answer: A

The correct answer is Osler-Rendu-Weber disease. All of this stuff is identifiable by the type of telangiectasia!! Know this: Linear telangiectasia on the face—actinically damaged skin; Broad telangiectasia—scleroderma associated with the CREST variant; Periungual telangiectasia—SLE, scleroderma, dermatomyositis; spider-like telangiectasia—Osler-Rendu-Weber disease.

488. Answer: D

The correct answer is syphilis. He has a classic rash of secondary syphilis. The palm and sole involvement is the classic "hallmark" for this disease. Chancre is commonly on the penis, but depending upon sexual practices, it can be on the pharynx or anus.

489. Answer: C

The correct answer is folate deficiency. He has vitiligo, which are macules that are completely lacking in pigment. It is generally a hereditary condition. Most cases are not associated with other disease processes; however, those listed besides folate deficiency have been described with this condition.

490. Answer: E

The correct answer is methyldopa. She has signs and symptoms of preeclampsia with increased BP and edema. She does not have headache or neurologic findings. She needs to be treated with an antihypertensive agent. In pregnancy, there is good data to show what NOT to use: ACE inhibitors and Nitroprusside should not be used. Other drugs to avoid include isotretinoin (Accutane), benzodiazepines, quinolones, tetracyclines, and warfarin.

491. Answer: B

The correct answer is IV heparin followed by subcutaneous heparin injections. Coumarin is absolutely contraindicated in pregnancy so all of the other answers should be thrown out. Thrombolytics would also be contraindicated. Heparin is also NOT without risks, but the risks are much greater that she will have recurrent pulmonary embolisms.

492. Answer: D

The correct answer is urine culture, HIV ELISA, and RPR. Most states require RPR testing and many are recommending that after proper counseling, HIV ELISA testing also be done. Urine culture is always done initially as asymptomatic bacteruria is quite common in pregnancy and these women have an increased risk of pyelonephritis and other infections. HSV II serology is essentially worthless. The main factor in determining if a woman is at risk for transmission of HSV is the presence of active lesions at the time of delivery—if present, then she would undergo a C-section.

493. Answer: C

The correct answer is to begin a trial of oral contraceptives. Irregular bleeding with intervals less than 18 days indicates a luteal phase abnormality. This can usually be alleviated with the use of oral contraceptives. If she had prolonged bleeding with normal intervals, then you would be concerned about submucosal fibroids. Other factors to consider in excessive or abnormal bleeding are spontaneous abortion or ectopic pregnancy. Medical causes of dysfunctional bleeding include hypothyroidism (doesn't this do just about everything??), liver disease with resultant coagulopathy, thrombocytopenia, and chronic renal failure.

494. Answer: C

The correct answer is endocervical polyp. Of those things listed, this is the most likely anatomic abnormality. Frequently, though, the examination will be normal.

495. Answer: E

The correct answer is endometriosis. Patients usually are nulliparous and over 30 with the following symptoms: dysmenorrhea, dyspareunia, dyschezia, and/or perimenstrual spotting. The most common site is the ovaries (look for tender adnexa in an afebrile patient).

496. Answer: A

The correct answer is serum pregnancy test. DON'T FORGET THAT PREGNANCY IS A COMMON PRESENTATION FOR PRIMARY AMENORRHEA IN TEENAGERS!!!! Teen pregnancy is a rampant problem in the U.S. and primary amenorrhea will commonly present this way! Don't forget it for the Boards!!

497. Answer: B

The correct answer is semen analysis. Here the answer is to go for cheap, easy, and relatively noninvasive. Infertility is a "male" problem a third of the time. Normal semen has the following properties: ejaculate volume >1ml; Sperm concentration > 20 million/ml; initial forward motility: >50% of sperm; Normal morphology >60% of sperm. I don't think the ABIM will ask this last stuff, except that they may ask about the concentration—but they would give you the normal values to figure out that the man was low on ammunition.

498. Answer: D

The correct answer is to continue with current regimen. This woman has HIV disease and had a low CD4 count and high viral load before starting on highly active antiretroviral therapy. The correct approach is to continue treating the patient with a very active regimen (three-drug therapy). This will keep the woman with the best immune system and keep the chance of transmission to the baby minimal (likely 1% or less). Zidovudine alone has been studied and lowers transmission rate from about 30% without antiretrovirals to 8% on zidovudine. Single drug therapy with zidovudine would not be appropriate because resistance would likely form and it would not protect the woman's immune system as well as her current regimen. It is also not as effective in reducing transmission as a three-drug regimen. There is no reason to switch to a different, potentially more toxic regimen (DDI/D4T/Amprenavir). Case reports of lactic acidosis occurring during pregnancy have been reported in women on D4T. The combination of D4T and DDI increases the risk of neuropathy in the patient.

499. Answer: C

The correct answer is to continue on OCP, intensify insulin regimen for target glycated Hb 6.0. This woman with type 1 DM wishes to become pregnant. She should have tight control of her diabetes during pregnancy, and it's especially important during the 1st trimester. She should work intensively at lowering her glycated Hb *before* getting pregnant. Target glycated Hb is 6.0.

500. Answer: B

The correct answer is to recommend Kegel exercises. This patient has symptoms typical of stress incontinence (episodes occurring when she laughs, sneezes, or coughs). Medications rarely work for this kind of incontinence. Kegel exercises are exercises where patients strengthen the pelvic floor muscles, which can help with urethral control of urine flow. Some patients with stress incontinence may need surgery to reposition the bladder.

501. Answer: C

The correct answer is *Bacillus cereus*. Let's "be serious" for a moment (Oooooo)…This is an obvious emergency and this organism is a bad one. It is associated with a penetrating injury to the eyeball. Remember also that it causes food poisoning, particularly the "Chinese rice-bowl" variety. *Acanthamoeba* is associated with contact lenses and solutions. *Staphylococcus epidermidis*—think about after ocular surgery—is usually present in particular with cataract extraction or lens implantation. It can also occur after trauma, but *B. cereus* is one of the few that will give you a ring abscess (*Pseudomonas* and *Proteus* are about the only other two). *Bartonella henselae*—no kitties around in the history and usually you'll get a conjunctivitis picture, …NOT this nasty scenario. So just remember: penetrating eye injury with ring abscess formation in the cornea: *B. cereus*! No really, I'm not kidding!

502. Answer: D

The correct answer is carotid duplex. This patient has the sudden onset of right eye visual loss. He has a history of diabetes but no history of retinopathy or evidence of retinopathy on the funduscopic exam. The diabetes is a major risk for vascular disease; the funduscopic finding of a "cherry red spot" is consistent with retinal artery occlusion. The most likely cause of this would be atherosclerotic plaque emboli from a diseased carotid artery. The most appropriate first diagnostic test would be a carotid duplex. If surgery is possible based on results of duplex, a carotid angiogram would be a reasonable secondary test prior to an endarterectomy. Head CT scan or MRI would not be diagnostically helpful in this case.

503. Answer: B

The correct answer is pituitary tumor. Chiasmal lesions interrupt the central fibers that mediate temporal vision—therefore, a pituitary tumor or craniopharyngioma results in loss of visual fields in the bitemporal regions. If the lesion was posterior to the chiasm—such as loss of visual cortex in one occipital lobe—a complete loss of visual perception in one field would result.

504. Answer: E

The correct answer is left sympathetic chain. The symptoms are consistent with sympathetic denervation of her left eye—the "Horner" pupil. Most commonly, pulmonary neoplasms of the superior sulcus will produce this lesion. Usually it is associated with ipsilateral ptosis and anhidrosis. Pupillary light responses should be normal, as should the response to agents that dilate and constrict the pupil. However, since the sympathetic chain is not working, cocaine cannot cause local release of sympathomimetic substances and is a poor dilator.

505. Answer: A

The correct answer is tonometry. He has acute angle-closure glaucoma. This has resulted in the obstruction of outflow from the aqueous humor at the iris. The buildup of intraocular pressure can be measured and requires urgent treatment with hyperosmotic agents. Permanent treatment will require laser therapy or surgical iridotomy.

506. Answer: D

The correct answer is presbyopia. This is the normal aspect of aging that occurs between the ages of 40 and 50. The lens slowly loses its ability to accommodate for near vision. Patients usually need bifocals or reading glasses for near vision.

507. Answer: D

The correct answer is glaucoma. This patient has noticed some visual changes. On funduscopic exam she has a high cup to disc ratio suggestive of glaucoma. A normal cup to disc ratio is usually less than 1:2. The retinal exam does not show hemorrhages or exudates that would be expected in a patient with advanced hypertensive retinopathy. This patient is much younger (58) than is usually seen with macular degeneration.

508. Answer: B

The correct answer is HIV retinopathy. This patient with HIV disease presents without visual symptoms. On funduscopic exam he has cotton wool spots without hemorrhage, suggesting HIV retinopathy. His high CD4 count effectively rules out CMV retinitis (almost always seen with CD4 count less than 50) and toxoplasmosis (rare above CD4 count of 100). Cryptococcus and cryptosporidia rarely ever cause retinal lesions.

509. Answer: C

The correct answer is cytomegalovirus retinitis. This patient has advanced HIV disease with a very low CD_4 count (26). Almost all individuals who develop CMV retinitis have CD_4 counts less than 50. He has typical symptoms of CMV retinitis (floaters). His funduscopic exam shows large hemorrhages and exudates consistent with CMV retinitis. HIV retinopathy is asymptomatic, and on funduscopic exam, cotton wool spots are seen. Retinal TB is much less common than CMV, and would be even less likely with the patient on active antituberculous therapy. Cryptococcus rarely ever involves the retina. Toxoplasmosis is a possibility but is far less common than CMV retinitis.

510. Answer: B

The correct answer is that it can be a very effective treatment of bipolar affective disorder. It is not a drug of choice for most major depressive disorders. It has many drug-drug interactions and the patient should be informed to notify all prescribers of medications that he is on Lithium. Lithium intoxication manifests as depression of mental status. Hypothyroidism is a potential side effect of the drug as it inhibits secretion of thyroid hormone.

511. Answer: A

The correct answer is good premorbid functioning. It is the best indictor of good prognosis. All of the other factors listed are actually predictors of poor prognosis.

512. Answer: C

The correct answer is antipsychotic medications and psychosocial treatment. Hopefully, this was an easy one for you. If this book is talking to you and telling you things right now, maybe you need to look into the correct answer for this question.

513. Answer: D

The correct answer is to give diphenhydramine or benztropine immediately. He is having an acute dystonic reaction. This usually occurs in the first hours or days of treatment. It is most common in younger men. The symptoms will improve rapidly with treatment.

514. Answer: E

The correct answer is all of the statements are true. KNOW THIS!! Men COMMIT suicide more often than women BUT women ATTEMPT suicide more often than men. Additional risk factors on the boards to look out for include history of alcohol or substance abuse, history of violence, prior psychiatric history, and recent major life change (separation, loss of job, etc.).

515. Answer: A

The correct answer is voluntary hospitalization unless he refuses then institute involuntary commitment. This man has made out a plan of action and has considered it in the last 24 hours. He needs to be hospitalized for his own protection at this point. It is not pertinent that he is "ok" now. He has a past history of suicide attempt and yesterday he was actually making a plan to proceed with another attempt.

516. Answer: E

The correct answer is all items listed are helpful clues. Be wary of the elderly patient with many of the symptoms/findings listed here. Particularly be aware of anhedonia (loss of pleasure from activities that usually bring pleasure—you know, like playing checkers at the bus stop or pulling grey hairs out of your knuckles—um..maybe this psych section is getting to me?).

517. Answer: C

The correct answer is adjustment disorder with depressed mood. Look for this when "a bad thing happens" on the Boards. The patient then cannot handle it well and feels malaise or a sense of things not right, etc. They generally do not meet the criteria for "full-blown" depression.

518. Answer: B

The correct answer is buspirone. It is non-addictive and non-sedating. A benzodiazepine could be used, but they are addictive and sedating.

519. Answer: E

The correct answer is Beta-amyloid protein. On a neuropathological level the disease is characterized by neurofibrillary tangles, which may contain an abnormally phosphorylated form of a microtubular protein as well as spherical deposits known as senile plaques. These plaques are made up of beta-amyloid protein.

520. Answer: B

The correct answer is paroxetine. Imipramine historically has been a good choice for panic disorder, which this woman has. The other agents are not effective for panic disorder.

521. Answer: A

The correct answer is to reduce the dose of chlorpromazine. He has tardive dyskinesia—manifested by his tongue thrusting and lip smacking gestures. Postural dystonia can also be part of this syndrome. The best thing to do is reduce the dose of medication. The problem with this, of course, is that he may have worsening of his thought disorder—so you have to watch for that. Akathisia, which he doesn't have, is characterized by obligatory movement of the extremities and motor restlessness--it may respond to treatment with beta-blockers. Also some patients will develop extrapyramidal side effects with symptoms similar to Parkinson's disease—this may respond to therapy with benztropine.

522. Answer: C

The correct answer is after the patient responds to emergent therapy, they may develop profound amnesic psychosis. Wernicke's encephalopathy is a consequence of thiamine (vitamin B1) deficiency. It is most commonly seen in chronic alcoholics however, well-documented cases have occurred in those without any alcohol intake. The classic triad listed is rare. Always administer thiamine before glucose!!!!!!!!!!!! Glucose in the absence of thiamine will worsen the disease! Thiamine administration will relieve the ocular palsies within hours. The ataxia and encephalopathy will more slowly resolve; but frequently the encephalopathy will leave a marked defect in memory and learning known as Korsakoff's psychosis. The major sites of brain involvement include the thalamus, hypothalamus, midbrain, floor of the 4th ventricle, and the cerebellar vermis.

523. Answer: D

The correct "incorrect" answer is left inferior quadrantanopia. All of the other items are common in these patients with Wernicke's aphasia. You would expect to find a right superior quadrantanopia due to the proximity of the inferior optic radiation to Wernicke's area in the left temporal lobe. Wernicke's is due to a lesion in the posterior temporal gyrus of the dominant hemisphere.

524. Answer: D

The correct "incorrect" answer is ESR. Use of screening tests in dementia workups are generally controversial—except when the tests are simple and inexpensive and the etiology is a potentially reversible cause of dementia. The four other tests listed are easy to do and relatively inexpensive. They are helpful in ruling out infectious (RPR), metabolic (Lytes, vitamin B12), and endocrine (TSH) etiologies for dementia. The ESR is not a specific test helpful for defining a cause of dementia.

525. Answer: C

The correct answer is obsessive-compulsive disorder. This disorder frequently begins in adolescence or early adulthood. Note the excessive handwashing and "door checking" – this is classic for this disorder. Treatment with selective serotonin reuptake inhibitors (SSRIs) or clomipramine may be effective.

526. Answer: A

The correct answer is benazepril/lithium interaction. This patient presents with symptoms consistent with lithium toxicity (diarrhea, nausea, vomiting, and ataxia. On exam he has fasciculations, cogwheel rigidity, and hyperreflexia). He was recently started on benazepril for hypertension. All ACE inhibitors inhibit renal excretion of lithium. Cimetidine and Tegretol do not affect lithium levels.

527. Answer: C

The correct answer is sodium bicarbonate. Sodium bicarbonate helps by alleviating depression of the sodium-dependent channel. Naloxone is a treatment for narcotic overdose. Physostigmine and phenytoin are not effective.

528. Answer: E

The correct answer is N-acetylcysteine + activated charcoal. This patient has an acetaminophen overdose. Hepatotoxicity is less when the combination of N-acetylcysteine is combined with activated charcoal (25% hepatotoxicity with N-acetylcysteine alone vs 4% when it is combined with activated charcoal).

529. Answer: A

The correct answer is no further testing. This elderly patient is admitted for surgical treatment of hip fracture and develops delirium and fever postoperatively. She has a nonfocal exam and most importantly an abnormal UA, suggesting UTI as the cause of delirium. Nosocomial meningitis is extremely rare especially if the patient has not had a neurosurgical procedure. If the patient has evidence of infection (pneumonia, UTI, Skin), then treatment of the infection is the appropriate course. Workup of a CNS infection is not necessary unless no alternative site of infection is found. Delirium and mental status changes are very common in the elderly when they develop infections.

530. Answer: D

The correct answer is cyclosporine. Cyclosporine is one of the drugs that will increase serum uric acid. In this man, he has GOUT. This is a drug interaction question! Always look for drug interactions as a possibility on the ABIM. They like to ask these because they are SO common and usually induced by US! Other drugs that will increase serum uric acid include diuretics, niacin, and ethambutol/pyrazinamide.

531. Answer: B

The correct answer is doxycycline. Common photosensitivity medications include: tetracyclines, sulfonamides, hydrochlorothiazide, phenothiazines, griseofulvin, sparfloxacin, and other quinolones. From highest risk to lowest risk of the quinolones:

1. Sparfloxacin
2. Lomefloxacin
3. Nalidixic acid
4. Enoxacin
5. Ciprofloxacin
6. Norfloxacin
7. Levofloxacin
8. Trovafloxacin

532. Answer: C

The correct answer is adverse effect due to ciprofloxacin. Quinolones have been well documented to be associated with tendon rupture. Reports include the shoulders, hands, and Achilles tendons. The Achilles tendon is the most common site. It can occur anytime during the course of therapy and even after treatment.

533. Answer: B

The correct answer is methanol. Methanol and ethylene glycol are the only agents that will potentially give you both a metabolic as well as an osmotic gap.

534. Answer: A

The correct "incorrect" answer is amitriptyline. Serum levels are not helpful in the management of tricyclic antidepressant overdoses!

535. Answer: B

The correct answer is 33.3%. This question asks you to calculate the sensitivity of Hemoccult testing in a defined patient population. To calculate sensitivity, it is the number of patients with a positive Hemoccult who have cancer (true positives) divided by the number of all patients with colon cancer in the study (true positives *plus* false negatives). For this case it would be 12 (the number of patients with Hemoccult positive stool who have cancer) divided by 12 (those with heme positive stool and cancer) + 24 (those with cancer who had heme negative stool). 12/(12+24) = 12/36 = 1/3 = 33.3%.

536. Answer: D

The correct answer is 12.5%. Positive predictive value is obtained by taking true positives/(true positives + false positives). In this case, 25/(25+175) = 12.5%.

537. Answer: A

The correct answer is 98.9%. The negative predictive value is the true negatives divided by (false negatives + true negatives). In this case: 890/(10 +890) = 98.9%.

538. Answer: C

The correct answer is No. The key here is the 95% confidence interval. It crosses over 0. This indicates that the differences between the new treatment and the standard therapy were NOT statistically significant. The numbers can be quite deceiving--even with such a large increase in survival. One possibility is that the study had too few patients to really have any power to show a significant difference between the two groups.

539. Answer: A

The correct answer is 5. Number of people needed to treat to prevent one bad outcome is based on 1/(absolute risk reduction) = 1/(the rate in the placebo group minus the rate in treatment group).
In our example: 1/(20/50 – 10/50) = 1/(.4-.2) = 1/(.2) = 5.

540. Answer: C

The correct answer is 71.4%. To calculate sensitivity you take true positives/(true positives + false negatives). In this case: 25/(25+10) = 71.4%.

541. Answer: B

The correct answer is 83.5%. To calculate specificity you take true negatives/(true negatives + false positives). In this case: 890/(890 + 175) = 83.5%.

542. Answer: D

The correct answer is the nephew's request to discontinue IVF and antibiotics is within his capacity to act as the patient's durable power of attorney for health care. Anytime someone has a durable power of attorney for HEALTH CARE—THEY RULE if the patient cannot make decisions for themselves.

543. Answer: E

The correct answer is do not give blood products. This patient has stated opinions against receiving blood products. This is confirmed by her husband. The overriding principle here is patient autonomy. She does not wish to receive blood products, and it is not appropriate for medical personnel to give blood products. If she were making a decision when she was not competent, then obtaining a representative for the patient would be appropriate.

544. Answer: B

The correct answer is treat with antibiotics because the patient has a life-threatening condition. This patient has a life-threatening condition (meningitis) that is likely affecting the patient's ability to make an informed decision. The patient has not refused medical care and has agreed to an invasive procedure (LP) but does not want antibiotics. You are not given information that the patient has a long-standing stance against medication (as seen with certain religions, e.g., Christian Science). The patient is somnolent and agitated when aroused, which is a change in baseline mental functioning. Because the patient has not demonstrated competency and is incapacitated by an acute illness, it is appropriate as the physician to intervene in the best interest of the patient. If a family member were present, then discussing it with them would be appropriate. A roommate has less decision-making authority in this case than the physician. Court orders are not practical in urgent situations like meningitis.

545. Answer: A

The correct answer is do not intubate the patient; keep him comfortable. This patient has clearly stated his wishes to not be intubated in the event of worsening pulmonary disease. He was competent at the time of the decision, and by not intubating him, you are respecting his wishes. The children's desires do not supersede the patient's right to autonomy.

546. Answer: C

The correct answer is detrusor overactivity. This patient has typical symptoms of urge incontinence, that is, she gets the message to urinate but is unable to make it to the toilet in time. Urge incontinence is due to detrusor overactivity. None of the medications she is on cause incontinence. Common medications that can lead to incontinence are diuretics and anticholinergic medications.

547. Answer: D

The correct answer is terazosin. This 76-year-old man has typical symptoms of prostatic obstruction. It is likely due to BPH. He has a normal PSA. Given his advanced age he does not need an aggressive workup for prostate cancer. The best initial treatment for BPH would be terazosin. Finasteride is not as effective as terazosin and takes longer to be effective. If he had increasing symptoms despite medical therapy, then consideration for surgery would be reasonable.

548. Answer: C

The correct answer is vascular disease. This elderly patient has erectile dysfunction but normal libido. Testosterone deficiency is common in elderly men, but when it causes erectile dysfunction it usually also causes decrease in libido. SSRIs can cause sexual side effects in about 30% of patients, but these are usually decrease in interest and delayed orgasm, not erectile dysfunction. This patient is on a lipid-lowering medication, making vascular disease more likely (risk factors of age and hyperlipidemia).

549. Answer: B

The correct answer is intraurethral alprostadil. This patient has erectile dysfunction with a normal libido. The normal libido would make testosterone deficiency less likely. Testosterone replacement would be inappropriate without documented low testosterone levels. He should not receive sildenafil (Viagra) because he is taking daily nitrates. Nitrate use is a contraindication for the use of Viagra. A penile implant would not be an appropriate initial therapy for erectile dysfunction.

550. Answer: A

The correct answer is breast exam, mammogram, Pap smear, and flex sig. This patient has not had any medical care or screening for at least 12 years. She should have Pap smear testing because she has not been screened for many years (if ever). It is appropriate not to do Pap testing in patients 65 or older if they are low risk (no new sexual partners and multiple prior normal Pap smears). She should have a mammogram and flexible sigmoidoscopy according to USPSTF and ACS guidelines.

551. Answer: D

The correct answer is cholesterol testing. This patient is 74 years old with Parkinson's disease and coronary artery disease. Prostate cancer screening is controversial. Even the most aggressive groups (ACS and AUA) only recommend it until 65-70 years of age. He should not get PSA testing (a slightly enlarged prostate is the norm for a 74 year old). Complete blood cell count is not an approved screening test. Cholesterol testing would be appropriate given his known CAD. Short-term and long-term benefits with cholesterol treatment in patients with CAD has been demonstrated.

552. Answer: B

The correct answer is Pneumovax, annual influenza, hep A series, and tetanus booster. Patients with HIV disease should receive an annual influenza vaccine and a Pneumovax every 6 years. This patient should also receive a hepatitis A series because of his hepatitis C infection. Hepatitis A can cause fatal hepatitis in hep C-infected individuals. A tetanus vaccine is appropriate, as he has not had one in over 10 years. He does not need a hepatitis B booster as he has serologic evidence of past hepatitis B infection.